Managing the Patient with Type II Diabetes

Andrew L. Wilson, PharmD, FASHP

Director
Pharmacy Services
Saint Louis University Hospital
St. Louis, Missouri

In Association with

Ila V. Mehra, PharmD, BCPS

Assistant Professor
Pharmacy Practice
Saint Louis College of Pharmacy
and Department of Family Medicine
Deaconess Hospital
St. Louis, Missouri

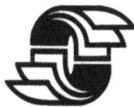

AN ASPEN PUBLICATION®
Aspen Publishers, Inc.
Gaithersburg, Maryland
1997

The authors have made every effort to ensure the accuracy of the information herein. However, appropriate information sources should be consulted, especially for new or unfamiliar procedures. It is the responsibility of every practitioner to evaluate the appropriateness of a particular opinion in the context of actual clinical situations and with due considerations to new developments. Authors, editors, and the publisher cannot be held responsible for any typographical or other errors found in this book.

With the exception of Chapters 13, 14, and 15, all material was originally published in *Pharmacy Practice Management Quarterly* issues 17:2 and 17:3.

Library of Congress Cataloging-in-Publication Data

Managing the patient with type II diabetes/[edited by] Andrew L.
Wilson, in association with Ila V. Mehra.
p. cm.
Includes bibliographical references and index.
ISBN 0-8342-1018-5
1. Non-insulin-dependent diabetes—Treatment. I. Wilson, Andrew
L. II. Mehra, Ila V.
[DNLM: 1. Diabetes Mellitus, Non-Insulin-Dependent—therapy—
collected works. WK 815 M266 1997]
RC662.18.M35 1997
616.4'6206—dc21
DNLM/DLC
for Library of Congress
97-23911
CIP

Orders: (800) 638-8437
Customer Service: (800) 234-1660

About Aspen Publishers • For more than 35 years, Aspen has been a leading professional publisher in a variety of disciplines. Aspen's vast information resources are available in both print and electronic formats. We are committed to providing the highest quality information available in the most appropriate format for our customers. Visit Aspen's Internet site for more information resources, directories, articles, and a searchable version of Aspen's full catalog, including the most recent publications: **http://www.aspenpub.com**
Aspen Publishers, Inc. • The hallmark of quality in publishing
Member of the worldwide Wolters Kluwer group.

Editorial Resources: Ruth Bloom
Library of Congress Catalog Card Number: 97-23911
ISBN: 0-8342-1018-5

Printed in the United States of America

1 2 3 4 5

Table of Contents

Contributors v

Preface vii

PART I—PATIENT MANAGEMENT STRATEGIES 1

Chapter 1— Strategies for the Treatment of Type II Diabetes Mellitus 3
    Ila V. Mehra

Chapter 2— Important Aspects of Self-Management Education in Patients
          with Diabetes 13
    Darren M. Stam and John P. Graham

Chapter 3— Approach to the Treatment of Diabetic Nephropathy 25
    John M. Burke

Chapter 4— Managing the Care of the Diabetic Transplant Patient 33
    Jerry Siegel, Victoria S. DeVore, and Sue M. Bosley

Chapter 5— Applying the Principles of Pharmaceutical Care to the Patient
          with Diabetes 43
    Richard Segal

PART II—DRUG THERAPY OF TYPE II DIABETES MELLITUS 49

Chapter 6— Exploring the Role of Sulfonylureas in the Treatment of
          Non–Insulin-Dependent Diabetes Mellitus 51
    John P. Graham and Darren M. Stam

Chapter 7— New Therapeutic Options in the Treatment of Diabetes Mellitus 59
    Cheryl Kentch Miller

Chapter 8— Managing Therapy and Adverse Effects with Antihyperglycemic
          Agents: A Focus on Metformin and Acarbose 69
          Beth Bryles Phillips

PART III—SUPPORTIVE THERAPY AND TREATMENT CONCERNS 79

Chapter 9— The Importance of the Pharmacist's Expanding Role on the
          Diabetes Team: Reinforcing Nutritional Guidelines for
          Improved Glycemic Control 81
          Linda C. Johnson and Elizabeth Beach

Chapter 10—Treatment of Hypertension in Patients with Diabetes................................... 93
          Bradley G. Phillips

Chapter 11—Issues in Treating the Geriatric Patient with Diabetes................................. 103
          Gordon A. Ireland

Chapter 12—Systematic Approach to the Management of the Type II
          Diabetic Patient: Case Presentation 111
          Lenore T. Coleman

PART IV—DISEASE MANAGEMENT AND ECONOMICS 121

Chapter 13—Disease State Management in Diabetes Care 123
          Catherine E. Cooke

Chapter 14—Are Pharmacists and Pharmaceutical Care Having an Impact
          on Diabetes? 129
          Maura F. Monaghan and Michael S. Monaghan

Chapter 15—Economic Evaluations and Diabetes 137
          Dev S. Pathak and Thomas A. Burke

Index 145

Contributors

Elizabeth Beach, MS, RD
Clinical Dietitian
St. Anthony's Medical Center
St. Louis, Missouri

Sue M. Bosley, PharmD
Pharmacy Practice Resident
Department of Pharmacy
The Ohio State University Medical Center
Columbus, Ohio

Thomas A. Burke, PharmD
Glaxo-Wellcome Pharmacoeconomics Fellow
The Ohio State University College of
  Pharmacy
Columbus, Ohio

John M. Burke, PharmD, BCPS
Associate Professor of Pharmacy Practice
Saint Louis College of Pharmacy
Department of Family Medicine
Deaconess Hospital
St. Louis, Missouri

Lenore T. Coleman, PharmD, CDE, FASHP
Health Care Support Specialist
Bayer Corporation
Altadena, California

Catherine E. Cooke, PharmD
Assistant Professor
Department of Pharmacy Practice and Science
University of Maryland at Baltimore
Baltimore, Maryland

Victoria S. DeVore, PharmD
Specialty Practice Resident in Renal/Internal
  Medicine
Department of Pharmacy
The Ohio State University Medical Center
Columbus, Ohio

John P. Graham, PharmD
Assistant Professor of Pharmacy Practice
Saint Louis College of Pharmacy
John Cochran VA Medical Center
St. Louis, Missouri

Gordon A. Ireland, PharmD
Associate Professor of Pharmacy Practice
St. Louis College of Pharmacy
The Veterans Affairs Medical Center of St.
  Louis
Adjunct Associate Professor of Medicine
Division of Geriatrics
St. Louis University Medical School
St. Louis, Missouri

Linda C. Johnson, RN, MS, CDE
Certified Diabetes Educator
West County Internal Medicine
St. Louis, Missouri

Ila V. Mehra, PharmD
Assistant Professor of Pharmacy Practice
Saint Louis College of Pharmacy
St. Louis, Missouri

Cheryl Kentch Miller, PharmD
Executive Director, Clinics
SCIREX Corporations
Hartford, Connecticut

David W. Miller, RPh, PhD
International Director
Department of Pharmacoeconomic Research
GlaxoWellcome Research and Development
Greenford, Middlesex ENGLAND

Maura J. Monaghan, PharmD, MBA
Clinical Services Manager, Pharmaceutical
    Services
Health Care Maintenance Operations
Mutual of Omaha Insurance Company
Omaha, Nebraska

Michael S. Monaghan, PharmD
Associate Professor
Department of Pharmacy Practice
Creighton University School of Pharmacy and
    Allied Health Professions
Omaha, Nebraska

Dev S. Pathak, DBA
Merrell Dow Professor
The Ohio State University College of
    Pharmacy
Columbus, Ohio

Beth Bryles Phillips, PharmD
Clinical Pharmacist, Ambulatory Care
Department of Pharmaceutical Care
University of Iowa Hospitals and Clinics
Iowa City, Iowa

Bradley G. Phillips, PharmD
Assistant Professor
University of Iowa College of Pharmacy
Division of Administrative Pharmacy
Iowa City, Iowa

Richard Segal, PhD
Professor and Chairman
Pharmacy Health Care Administration
University of Florida
Gainesville, Florida

Jerry Siegel, RPh, FASHP
Senior Director, Pharmaceutical Services
The Ohio State University Medical Center
Columbus, Ohio

Darren M. Stam, PharmD
Assistant Professor of Pharmacy Practice
Saint Louis College of Pharmacy
John Cochran VA Medical Center
St. Louis, Missouri

Preface

Chronic diseases continue to plague humanity, even as we make progress in treating acute illness. Asthma, congestive heart failure, hypertension, and diabetes mellitus, among others, continue to have serious impact on life span, quality of life, and health care costs in the United States. When considering the impact of disease on the public health, diabetes mellitus has moved to the forefront for several reasons. First, adult onset (type II) diabetes appears to be increasing in prevalence in the United States. This increase may result from diet, lifestyle, or other human and environmental factors. This increase in prevalence magnifies the societal impact of the disease.

Second, type II diabetes causes a slow degenerative effect on nearly all body systems. It exacts a personal toll by causing or exacerbating cardiac, circulatory, neurologic, and degenerative diseases, extending their impact and increasing the speed of their progression. The indirect personal and societal costs of type II diabetes mellitus are increased by a degree of magnitude when considered under this rubric. It is the rare patient with diabetes who does not experience some real life-changing effect of the disease or its sequelae.

Third, the impact and progression of type II diabetes mellitus can be ameliorated only through the combined efforts of all members of the health care team. More than many acute and chronic diseases, Type II diabetes mellitus requires the combined resources of physicians in a number of specialties, nurses, dietitians, and pharmacists and, most importantly, the involvement of the patient and his or her family.

Fourth, new drugs and monitoring devices, alone or combined with existing therapies in disease management strategies, offer new therapeutic opportunities. Outcomes-based assessment of the success and impact of multidisciplinary strategies offers the ability to draw more robust and far-reaching conclusions and to apply them effectively to all patients.

Finally, the growing emphasis on cost containment has moved diabetes to a prominent place in the activities of managed care organizations. Due to the nature of the disease, patients with diabetes consume far greater amounts of direct health care dollars when compared with like patients without diabetes. Diabetic patients make more physician visits and are hospitalized more frequently than the general population. They use more drugs and are subject to a higher incidence of adverse drug reactions and therapeutic reverses and failures. Strategies designed to refine the delivery of care to patients with diabetes and to increase the effectiveness of therapeutic interventions can have a large impact on the financial success of health plans.

This text has a wide reach. It is designed to assist pharmacy students, practitioners, and managers in understanding the current state of care and management of the type II diabetic patient. It offers perspectives on overall patient care strategy; the place of pharmaceutical care in diabetes care; drug therapy, including newer agents, and strategies managing the patient who has complications of diabetes. Chapters also address diet and nutrition, patient education, health care team involvement, disease management, and the economics of treatment. The book is divided into four sections: *Patient Management Strategies, Drug Therapy of Type II Diabetes Mellitus, Supportive Therapy and Treatment Concerns,* and *Disease Management and Economics.* Each section offers a spectrum of information and ideas about issues in the treatment of type II diabetes mellitus.

I acknowledge each of the authors for their contribution to this text. Their practice skills and knowledge are evidenced in their contributions. Ila Mehra deserves special recognition for her guidance and editing of the original articles as they appeared in *Pharmacy Practice Management Quarterly.* Dr. Mehra's personal interest, skill, and perseverance saw the project through from its initial phases. I also thank Uday Jodhpurkar of Bayer Pharmaceuticals for his personal and professional support.

Andrew L. Wilson, Pharm.D., FASHP
Editor

Since the original development of the manuscript, The American Diabetes Association (ADA) has revised the guidelines for assigning the diagnosis of diabetes mellitus (DM). A patient demonstrating any one of the three criteria listed below is considered to have demonstrated the presence of active DM:

- Symptoms of DM and a random plasma glucose of > 200 mg/dl
- A fasting plasma glucose of > 126 mg/dl
- A 2-hour postprandial glucose of > 200 mg/dl during an oral glucose tolerance test (75 g).

Patients with a fasting plasma glucose of 100–125 mg/dl are considered to have impaired fasting glucose. Impaired glucose tolerance is defined as a 2 hour postprandial glucose of 140–199 mg/dl. More frequent testing is indicated if risk factors and/or either impaired fasting glucose or impaired glucose tolerance is present.

(Source: *Diabetes Care.* 1997;20:1183–1197)

Patient Management Strategies

Type II diabetes mellitus is a chronic debilitating disease with many differing and far-reaching effects. The manifestations of the disease are different in each patient, and the patient's and family's ability to provide support also varies. For these reasons, and the expected variation in patient response to treatment, the success of treatment hinges on a coherent and thoughtful patient management plan.

An effective patient management plan is current, using recent data and information to develop and implement a core treatment strategy. Drugs, monitoring devices and regimens, diet, and supportive care are all synthesized to achieve the greatest results. Many issues, such as the desirable degrees of glycemic control and the selection and combination of pharmaceuticals, are controversial and subject to changes as outcome data accumulate. Ila Mehra provides a current prospective on the selection of an overall strategy, including an understanding of pathogenesis of the disease, the initiation of drug therapy, and selection of drugs. Dr. Mehra also addresses the issue of tight control, although the jury is still out on the effectiveness of fastidious glucose management.

Patient involvement is critical to treatment success. This truism is accentuated in chronic disease and is even more crucial to a disease such as diabetes in which diet, exercise, and daily monitoring play a large role in therapy.

The American Diabetes Association has identified patient education and understanding of the disease and its therapy as the cornerstone of successful management. Stam and Graham identify and elucidate key factors in patient self-management. The pharmacist's role in self-management is the education of the patient and the development of skills and awareness necessary to achieve the goals of therapy.

Chapters by Burke and by Siegel, DeVore, and Bosley describe therapeutic issues in dealing with a common complication of diabetes, nephropathy and kidney failure. Successful treatment of the underlying disease often delays or ameliorates the onset of this complication and the resulting dialysis and kidney transplantation. However, equally important to long-term success, the underlying diabetes mellitus must continue to be a focus. The authors focus on the aspects of diabetes care that are unique to patients with advanced renal complications and kidney transplant.

Finally, Richard Segal synthesizes the larger roles of the pharmacist under the umbrella of pharmaceutical care. This powerful concept finds a place in the care of the diabetes patient. Pharmacists who accept a more global approach to accountability for medication therapy can improve the quality of life and the success of treatment of patients under their care. Dr. Segal provides concrete examples and guidance for implementing this philosophy of care.

CHAPTER 1

Strategies for the Treatment of Type II Diabetes Mellitus

Ila V. Mehra, PharmD, BCPS

In Type II diabetes mellitus (DM), the two primary defects that occur are insulin resistance and impaired insulin secretion. Currently, no data exist showing improved outcomes or reduced macrovascular complications with tight glycemic control in Type II DM, and only minimal data show a reduction of microvascular complications. Still, the current standard of practice is to attempt to attain glycemic goals in patients with Type II DM. As an attempt to resolve this issue, the United Kingdom Prospective Diabetes Study (UKPDS) was initiated. This 11-year study is comparing conventional therapy to intensive therapy in patients with Type II DM. The American Diabetes Association's (ADA) guidelines state that either sulfonylureas, metformin, acarbose, or insulin can be used as first-line treatment for Type II DM; however, oral agents can be attempted first in most patients. Until results from the ongoing UKPDS trials are available, the guidelines for glycemic control from the ADA should be followed. Key words: *acarbose, combination, drug therapy, insulin, metformin, sulfonylureas, Type II diabetes mellitus*

Until recently, the pharmacotherapy of Type II diabetes mellitus (DM) was limited to sulfonylureas (SUs) and insulin. When patients failed SU therapy, which was inevitable in time, they were switched to insulin or put on combination therapy. Those patients who refused insulin or were unable to take it, had no other alternative but to live with uncontrolled blood sugars and the symptoms and complications of poor glycemic control. Fortunately, new hope for patients with Type II DM arose a couple of years ago with the availability of new oral agents with different mechanisms of action than SUs. Metformin and acarbose provide new options in the treatment of Type II DM and may be used as monotherapy or in combination with SUs or insulin. Troglitazone is also now available; however, it was approved after this article was written and is not included.

The availability of metformin and acarbose not only offers diversity, but also confusion, in drug therapy selection. When a patient is first diagnosed with Type II DM and fails nonpharmacologic therapy, the clinician now has a choice of which oral agent to prescribe. Which drug should be used as initial therapy? Can therapy be individualized? Does "tight" glycemic control prevent complications in Type II DM? Do differences in efficacy exist between the agents? When one drug fails, which combination(s) of drug therapy should be used? These questions must be answered before clinicians can make the best use of the oral agents and insulin available for diabetes to provide improved quality of life and, hopefully, better outcomes for patients.

The author thanks Terry Seaton, PharmD, BCPS for helpful review of this manuscript.

PATHOGENESIS

Before appropriate drug therapy can be selected, an understanding of the pathogenesis of Type II diabetes is necessary. The two primary defects that occur are insulin resistance and impaired insulin secretion.[1] Resistance to the effects of insulin occurs in the skeletal muscle, liver, and adipose tissue, which leads to impaired glucose utilization, an inappropriate increase in hepatic gluconeogenesis, and lipolysis. Because of the uncontrolled hepatic glucose production that insulin no longer can control, fasting hyperglycemia ensues. Despite hyperinsulinemia, the increase in circulating insulin is insufficient to reduce the plasma glucose.[1]

Insulin deficiency also contributes to the development of Type II DM and may occur after insulin resistance. It has been hypothesized that insulin resistance occurs very early in the development of Type II DM, followed by an increase of insulin secretion from pancreatic beta cells to compensate and maintain normal glucose concentrations. When the beta cells cannot maintain this hypersecretion of insulin, a "relative deficiency" of insulin leads to impaired glucose tolerance, followed by clinical diabetes.[2]

While it is known that both insulin resistance and impaired insulin secretion occur, the issue of "which came first" is still hotly debated.[1-3] Although one large study [4] and many smaller studies [5] in persons with first-degree relatives with Type II DM support the insulin resistance theory, equal data exist to the contrary.[5] A large genetic study and numerous smaller studies in similar patient populations support the theory that insulin deficiency is the primary defect in the development of Type II DM.[5] Problems with study design have brought about questions of the validity of many of these studies.[5] More genetic studies will hopefully resolve the issue.

Probably one of the greatest controversies in Type II DM is the issue of hyperinsulinemia and its consequences. It is known that patients with Type II DM often present with insulin resistance syndrome (previously called "syndrome X"), which relates hyperinsulinemia with diabetes, obesity, hypertension, and hyperlipidemia. Abdominal obesity can increase the risk of hyperinsulinemia, which can lead to hypertension (through sodium retention, vascular hypertrophy, renin secretion, and sympathetic nervous system activation), hyperlipidemia, and impaired fibrinolysis.[6-8] These factors are thought to contribute to the macrovascular complications of diabetes such as coronary, cerebrovascular, and peripheral vascular disease, which are major causes of morbidity and mortality in patients with Type II DM. Evidence exists to support the association between hyperinsulinemia, rather than hyperglycemia, and macrovascular disease in Type II DM.

First, it has been shown that tight glycemic control decreases microvascular complications in patients with Type I DM[9]; however, it is unknown if glycemic control reduces macrovascular complications in either Type I or Type II DM. Second, the incidence of vascular events has been shown to increase very early in the course of the disease and has been seen before overt diabetes with chronic hyperglycemia develops.[10] Third, studies have demonstrated an association between hyperinsulinemia and an elevated risk of coronary heart disease (CHD).[11-13]

Even after controlling for potential confounding factors, hyperinsulinemia was shown to be an independent risk factor for the development of ischemic heart disease in patients without diabetes in the Quebec Cardiovascular Study.[14] In addition, a cohort study showed that the presence of both hyperinsulinemia and microalbuminuria was a strong risk factor for CHD events and CHD deaths in elderly nondiabetic individuals, even after controlling for other risk factors.[15] However, no prospective data exist to show a reduction of macrovascular disease if insulin sensitivity is improved or insulin levels are lowered. To add to the controversy, other reports have not shown an association between hyperinsulinemia and increased incidence of CHD.[10,16] In addition, controversy still exists as to the significance of exogenous insulin versus endogenous insulin to the contribution of CHD risk.

INITIATION OF DRUG THERAPY

Lifestyle modifications should be attempted first for three months and continued indefinitely.[10] Pharmacologic therapy should then be initiated if glycemic goals are not attained. If the patient is motivated and follows a diet and exercise plan, often drug therapy may be delayed. Mazze and associates have recommended that drug therapy with SUs be started at the time of diagnosis of Type II DM if a random blood glucose (RBG) is greater than 250 mg/dl or a fasting blood glucose (FBG) is 200–300 mg/dl.[17] Insulin should be considered at diagnosis if an RBG is greater than 450 mg/dl or if an FBG is greater than 300 mg/dl with hyperglycemic symptoms, or if the patient has an acute intercurrent illness or ketosis.[17]

TIGHT CONTROL IN TYPE II DM?

Clinicians strive for "tight glycemic control" in their patients with Type II DM, and the American Diabetes Association (ADA) recommends fairly tight glycemic goals (HbA$_{1c}$ of less than 7%, FBG 80–120 mg/dl)[10] in these patients. While the landmark Diabetes Control and Complications Trial (DCCT) resulted in a reduced progression of microvascular complications with tight glycemic control, only patients with Type I DM were evaluated.[9] Minimal data exists showing reduced macrovascular complications with tight glycemic control in Type II DM. One six-year trial in Japanese patients with Type II DM showed that tighter control with multiple daily insulin injections resulted in a decrease in the onset and progression of diabetic retinopathy, nephropathy (assessed by degree of albuminuria) and neuropathy (assessed by nerve conduction velocity) in comparison with conventional insulin therapy.[18] However, the trial was small (110 patients), was only in Japanese patients, did not control for factors such as ACE-inhibitor use, did not assess symptoms of neuropathy, and did not evaluate oral therapy. The University Group Diabetes Program (UGDP) did not demonstrate a reduction in diabetic complications after 11 years of improved glycemic control with SU, biguanide, or insulin therapy in patients with Type II DM.[19] This study has been criticized due to trial design. Currently, no data exist showing improved outcomes or decreased macrovascular complications with tight control in Type II DM. Still, the current standard of practice is to attempt to attain glycemic goals in patients with Type II DM.

The United Kingdom Prospective Diabetes Study

As an attempt to resolve this issue, the United Kingdom Prospective Diabetes Study (UKPDS) was initiated. This 11-year study is comparing conventional therapy (goal FBG < 270 mg/dl with no symptoms) to intensive therapy (goal FBG < 108 mg/dl) in patients with Type II DM. Six-[20] and nine-year[21] data have been published; study completion is expected in 1998.

The first endpoint being evaluated is diabetes-related mortality from myocardial infarction (MI), stroke, renal failure, sudden death, peripheral vascular disease (PVD) and/or amputations, and hypo- or hyperglycemic coma. The second endpoint is total mortality. The third endpoint is diabetes-related mortality and major clinical endpoints including nonfatal MI, angina with electrocardiogram (ECG) abnormality, heart failure, major stroke, amputation, retinopathy complications, and renal failure. Risk factors for complications including smoking, exercise, obesity, lipid subfractions, microalbuminuria, and blood pressure control are also being assessed.

The study consists of two separate comparisons. Conventional therapy with diet is being compared to intensive therapy with insulin and/or SU therapy in all patients; a separate arm in obese patients only is comparing conventional therapy with diet to intensive therapy with metformin, SUs, and/or insulin. If necessary, patients in the conventional therapy groups can be transferred to another therapy, and other oral agents and/or insulin can be added in the intensive therapy groups. There is no ceiling to the dose of insulin; doses can be increased infinitely.[20] Acarbose was added as a treatment option when it became available in 1994–1995, six years into the study.[19] The final results of the UKPDS will help to determine if intensive glycemic control will prevent either or both micro- and macrovascular complications in patients with Type II DM. Differences among therapies will also be evaluated.

Preliminary Study Results

At the end of nine years in the UKPDS, glycemic control (HbA1c) was significantly lower in the intensive group than the conventional group in both obese and nonobese patients (median 6.7% vs. 7.5%; p < 0.0001), as would be expected. The HbA1c surprisingly returned to baseline after approximately six years of intensive treatment regardless of the therapy, and continued to increase until it was greater than baseline, despite the fact that there was no ceiling to the dose of insulin.[21] This, again, raises the question: Is tight control possible in patients with Type II DM? The rate of increase of the HbA1c appeared to be lower in the last three years.[21] This may have been due, in part, to postprandial hyperglycemia that was contributing to the increase in HbA1c, which improved after the addition of acarbose for the last three years, or because of additional therapies added to prevent marked hyperglycemia.

Similarly, FBG was significantly lower with intensive treatment than conventional treatment (median 131 mg/dl vs. 162 mg/dl; p < 0.0001). After an initial decline, FBG gradually but steadily increased in both groups.[21] From years one to six, patients in the insulin group had significantly less of an increase in FBG than the SU group.[20]

At nine years, there was no difference in overall glycemic control between any of the therapies in the intensive treatment groups. Whether patients received SU, metformin, or high doses of insulin, glycemic control was similar, and worsened after an initial improvement.

In the UKPDS, intensive treatment with either SU or insulin resulted in significantly higher fasting insulin levels than conventional therapy. At six and nine years, the subgroup of obese patients receiving metformin had significantly lower fasting insulin levels than at baseline, and significantly lower insulin levels than conventional treatment and insulin/SU intensive treatment. Similar FBG with metformin and SU and/or insulin with lower insulin levels may suggest improved insulin sensitivity. Directly measured insulin sensitivity was also significantly higher in the metformin group at six years.[20,21] Although metformin improves insulin sensitivity and reduces insulin levels, no data are available yet to show a reduction in cardiovascular morbidity or mortality compared to agents that increase insulin.

After six and nine years of therapy, body weight was significantly higher with intensive therapy with SU or insulin than with conventional therapy, and the insulin group gained more weight than the SU group. Unexpectedly, there was no significant difference in body weight between metformin and diet at six and nine years.[20,21]

One potential limitation of the UKPDS is that different therapeutic agents may be added as glycemic control worsens. Therefore, it will be difficult to separate out the groups when the final data are analyzed. The nine-year data thus far show no significant difference in glycemic control or complications, regardless of the drug therapy used. Twenty percent of the study group as a whole had a macrovascular event and nine percent had a microvascular event. Glycemic control eventually worsened following an initial improvement. No differences have emerged yet between intensive treatment and conventional treatment, or between therapies. Acarbose has not yet been evaluated separately. When the final 11-year data are published, hopefully the question of the need for (or the possibility of) tight glycemic control in Type II DM will be answered. Until then, the ADA guidelines for glycemic control[10] should be followed.

WHICH AGENT FOR INITIAL THERAPY?

Although the degree of glycemic control in Type II DM has not been fully determined, drug therapy should be initiated within three months after beginning diet and exercise.[10] The ADA guidelines state that either SU, metformin, acarbose, or insulin can be used as first-line treatment for Type II DM. However, oral agents can be attempted first in most patients. Insulin results in the most weight gain and is cumbersome for patients. In addition, the potential for the consequences of worsened hyperinsulinemia and insulin resistance exist.

SUs are a rational first choice for many patients, especially for those who are not obese. SUs are effective (reduce HbA$_{1c}$ by 1½%–2%), inexpensive, have few side effects, and can often be taken once a day.[10] The most common side effects are weight gain and hypoglycemia.[22]

Metformin may be a good choice for first-line therapy in obese patients, and possibly those with hyperlipidemia and hypertension. Metformin results in similar glycemic control as SUs.

Studies have shown that metformin either decreases weight[23,24] or has no significant difference than diet alone,[7,21] while SU and insulin increase weight. Some data also show an improvement in hyperlipidemia; studies have shown a reduction in total cholesterol by 10 percent–18 percent, a lowering of triglycerides by 10 percent–20 percent (up to a 50% reduction in hypertriglyceridemic patients), and an increase in high density lipoprotein by 10 percent–28 percent.[24,25] Blood pressure was also reduced in patients with hypertension taking metformin.[25] In addition, metformin monotherapy reduces insulin concentration[21] and does not normally cause hypoglycemia.[26] Disadvantages include numerous contraindications, bothersome side effects (mostly gastrointestinal), two- to three-times-a-day dosing, and the potential for lactic acidosis.[26] No data are available showing a difference in outcomes between SU and metformin in the treatment of Type II DM. Ideally, the patient should be involved in the selection of initial drug therapy, by discussing the efficacy, adverse effects, and frequency of dosing.

Although acarbose mainly decreases postprandial glucose (PPG), some studies have shown a reduction in FBG. The reduction in PPG is approximately 50–60 mg/dl.[27,28] The improvement in overall glycemic control is generally less with

acarbose monotherapy (reduces HbA$_{1c}$ by ½%–1%) than with SU or metformin.[10] Postprandial insulin concentration, triglycerides (by about 20%) and weight may also decrease with acarbose.[23,29,30] Disadvantages include side effects (mostly gastrointestinal), three-times-a-day dosing, and the need for using glucose tablets for the treatment of hypoglycemic episodes.[29] As initial therapy, acarbose may be preferred in patients (especially obese) with significant postprandial hyperglycemia (PPG > 250 mg/dl), with FBG < 160–170, and/or mildly elevated HbA$_{1c}$. Details concerning adverse effects and management of therapy with metformin and acarbose are beyond the scope of this article.

AFTER FAILURE OF INITIAL THERAPY

Initial therapy should be continued for three to six months with continued diet and exercise. The dose should be titrated upward based on results of home blood glucose monitoring. Overall glycemic control should be assessed with an HbA$_{1c}$ to determine if the initial treatment is effective, before changing or adding therapy.

If glycemic control is not achieved or is eventually lost on initial therapy, attempts at improving glycemic control should be made. Figures 1 and 2 are proposed algorithms for therapy following treatment failures with SU and metformin, respectively. These algorithms are based on available data and, in the absence of clinical studies, opinion and anecdotal experience. These algorithms are general guidelines that are not patient-specific.

SU failure

Although changing to a different SU is generally not effective,[31] one crossover study in 132 patients showed that the controlled-release formulation of glipizide resulted in a significantly lower mean FBG than an equal dose of the immediate-release formulation after one and eight weeks of treatment. Although HbA$_{1c}$ was similar, it was assessed only after eight weeks of treatment; usually three months are necessary for accurate evaluation. Subanalyses showed

When initial therapy fails . . .

SULFONYLUREA FAILURE

No contraindications to metformin

Postprandial hyperglycemia

Contraindication to metformin and significant fasting hyperglycemia

ADD METFORMIN

Failure of combination

ADD ACARBOSE*

Failure of SU/acar combination

ADD INSULIN (if sig. fasting hyperglycemia) OR ADD ACARBOSE

Change to:
Insulin + SU OR
Insulin + metformin

Change to:
SU + METFORMIN

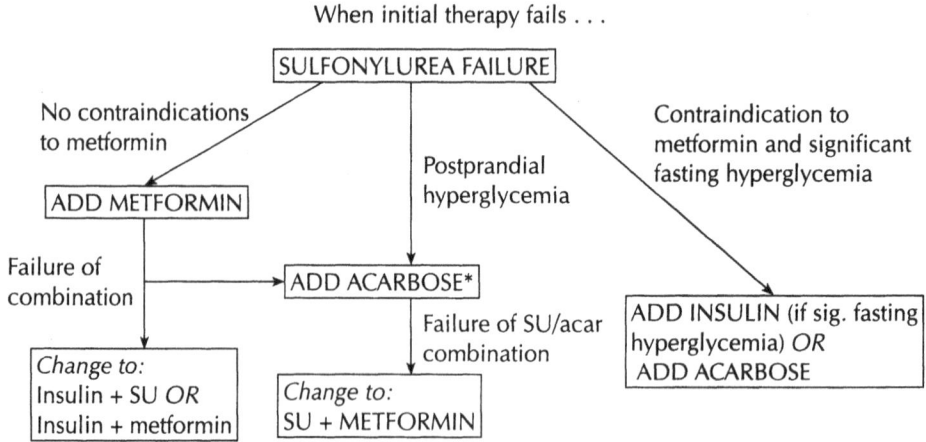

Figure 1. Proposed algorithm for treatment after initial failure of SU therapy.

that the difference was only significant in more poorly controlled patients with FBG > 198 mg/dl, and was associated with higher fasting glipizide concentrations in the controlled-release glipizide group.[32] This may be due to decreased absorption of immediate-release glipizide at higher plasma glucose levels. A small study in healthy volunteers showed that the absorption of immediate-release glipizide was decreased by 50 percent when the plasma glucose concentration was > 198 mg/dl after experimentally induced hyperglycemia.[33] The exact mechanism is unknown; however, hypergly-

cemia has been shown to impair gastric motility and emptying, possibly by increasing somatostatin secretion.[32] Therefore, a trial of controlled-release glipizide after primary SU failure with an immediate-release formulation is an option, especially in the face of significant hyperglycemia when impaired absorption is a possibility.

Patients who started on an SU and still have significant fasting hyperglycemia should add metformin if no contraindications exist. Adding metformin to SU has been shown to significantly reduce FBG and HbA$_{1c}$ (by 63 mg/dl and 1.7%,

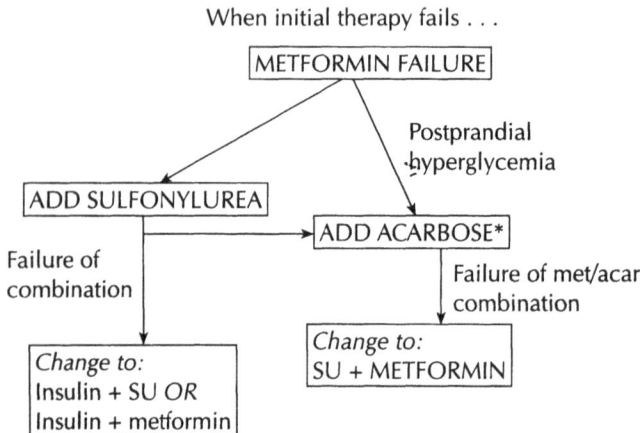

When initial therapy fails . . .

METFORMIN FAILURE

Postprandial hyperglycemia

ADD SULFONYLUREA

Failure of combination

ADD ACARBOSE*

Failure of met/acar combination

Change to:
Insulin + SU OR
Insulin + metformin

Change to:
SU + METFORMIN

Figure 2. Proposed algorithm for treatment after initial failure of metformin therapy.

respectively), whereas switching to metformin resulted in similar glycemic control than continuing glyburide.[34] In clinical studies, adding metformin to SU has resulted in a greater reduction in HbA1c than adding acarbose.[23] If the patient has significant postprandial hyperglycemia (PPG > 250 mg/dl), however, the next step may be to add acarbose. A small crossover study showed that adding acarbose to SU resulted in a significantly better reduction in two-hour PPG than adding metformin (146 mg/dl vs. 176 mg/dl; $p < 0.05$), while reaching similar reductions in FBG and HbA1c.[35] A larger study also showed a significant reduction in both FBG (by 25 mg/dl) and HbA1c (by 0.9%)when acarbose was added to SU.[36] Therefore, even if significant fasting hyperglycemia exists, adding acarbose is an option if the patient has a contraindication to metformin. However, insulin may eventually be necessary in many patients.

The combination of SU and insulin is a good option in patients who still have significant fasting hyperglycemia on maximum dose SU but have a contraindication to metformin. Although many different regimens exist, the most studied is morning SU and bedtime NPH insulin (BIDS). This combination results in an improved FBG and HbA1c. The main adverse effects of this combination are hypoglycemia, additive weight gain, and further increase in insulin concentration.[37]

Metformin failure

In patients who start with metformin and no longer have adequate glycemic control, the next rational step would be to add an SU. There are no data to support switching from metformin to SU. If the patient has significant postprandial hyperglycemia or is obese, an option would be to add acarbose; however, additive gastrointestinal side effects may limit the use of this combination. Although limited, data exist showing improved glycemic control when acarbose was added to metformin.[36] Acarbose may decrease the bioavailability of metformin when given concomitantly, although the clinical signifi-

cance of this interaction has not been determined.[10]

The combination of metformin and insulin is another option. The addition of metformin in poorly controlled patients with Type II DM taking insulin resulted in significant reductions in HbA1c and glucose profile, while allowing for a 25 percent reduction in the dose of insulin.[38] The newest insulin analog, lispro, is another option to add to either SU or metformin dosing three times a day before meals.[39]

Acarbose failure

For those patients started on acarbose, the addition of an SU would be reasonable, especially in nonobese patients. The combination of acarbose and metformin is another option in obese patients, if the patient can tolerate the adverse gastrointestinal effects. Another option would be to switch acarbose to SU or metformin, depending on current glycemic control and degree of fasting hyperglycemia.

Failure of dual combination therapy

Combination therapy should be given a trial of a minimum of three months, unless the patient has severe hyperglycemia or symptoms, and an HbA1c should confirm therapeutic failure. Two options are available if dual therapy fails: triple oral therapy or insulin with metformin. Triple combination oral therapy with SU, metformin, and acarbose is an option, although it has not been well studied. One small trial in 36 patients evaluated the addition of acarbose to poorly controlled patients taking either SU alone or SU and metformin for six months. The results showed a significant decrease in HbA1c, postprandial blood glucose, fasting triglycerides, and body weight.[30] Insulin in combination with two oral agents has not been studied, but may be attempted.

If patients fail combination oral therapy, a C-peptide concentration, which measures pancreatic insulin secretion, may be helpful to obtain to rule out the possibility of Type I DM or pancreatic "burn out." However, the usefulness of this test in this situation has not been evaluated.

Eventually, some patients may require insulin therapy alone. This is often used as last-line therapy because very high doses are sometimes needed, which can cause increased appetite, further weight gain, and further insulin resistance, which may necessitate higher insulin doses and contribute to the vicious cycle.[37] Insulin alone is recommended after failure of different dual combination therapies and/or triple therapy,[39] or in the presence of severe insulin deficiency manifesting with ketonuria and/or significant weight loss.

•   •   •

Two questions still exist concerning the treatment of Type II DM. First, is any one agent preferred over another? No statistically and/or clinically significant differences in long-term efficacy or outcomes have yet been shown between SU, metformin, acarbose, and insulin monotherapy in Type II DM. For now, effects on glucose control, weight, cholesterol, and blood pressure, as well as adverse effects, can help guide selection of patient-specific drug therapy. The proposed algorithms in Figures 1 and 2 can help guide the treatment approach once a patient fails initial therapy.

Second, how important is tight glycemic control in Type II DM? No data currently show that tight control improves outcomes or reduces diabetic macrovascular complications. Data showing reduced microvascular complications is minimal. For now, the guidelines for glycemic control from the ADA[10] should be followed.

When the UKPDS is completed, hopefully these questions will be answered. In addition, a six-year Veterans Affairs Cooperative Study is ongoing and is comparing standard insulin treatment (goal HbA$_{1c}$ about 9%) with intensive insulin treatment (goal HbA$_{1c}$ < 7.5%) in patients with Type II DM. The primary endpoint will be major cardiovascular events, and other endpoints are retinopathy, nephropathy, and neuropathy.[40] Until these trials are published, clinicians can only hope that good glycemic control will have some improvement in outcomes in patients with Type II DM.

REFERENCES

1. Taylor, S.I., Accili, D., and Imai Y. "Insulin Resistance or Insulin Deficiency: Which is the Primary Cause of NIDDM?" *Diabetes* 43 (1994): 735–40.

2. Polonsky, K.S., Sturis, J., and Bell, G.I. "Non–Insulin-Dependent Diabetes Mellitus: A Genetically Programmed Failure of the Beta Cell to Compensate for Insulin Resistance." *New England Journal of Medicine* 334, no.12 (1996): 777–83.

3. Weir, G.C. "Which Comes First in Non–Insulin-Dependent Diabetes Mellitus: Insulin Resistance or Beta-Cell Failure? Both Come First." (Editorial) *Journal of the American Medical Association* 273, no. 23 (1995): 1,878–79.

4. Warram, J., et al. "Slow Glucose Removal Rate and Hyperinsulinemia Precede the Development of Type II Diabetes in the Offspring of Diabetic Parents." *Annals of Internal Medicine* 113 (1990): 909–15.

5. Pimenta W., et al. "Pancreatic Beta-Cell Dysfunction as the Primary Genetic Lesion in NIDDM." *Journal of the American Medical Association* 273, no. 23 (1995): 1,855–61.

6. Kaplan, N.M. "The Deadly Quartet: Upper-Body Obesity, Glucose Intolerance, Hypertriglyceridemia, and Hypertension." *Archives of Internal Medicine* 149 (1989): 1,514–20.

7. DeFronzo, R.A. and Ferrannini, E. "Insulin Resistance: A Multifaceted Syndrome Responsible for NIDDM, Obesity, Hypertension, Dyslipidemia, and Atherosclerotic Cardiovascular Disease." *Diabetes Care* 14, no. 3 (1991): 173–94.

8. Stolar, M.W. "Atherosclerosis in Diabetes: The Role of Hyperinsulinemia." *Metabolism* 37, no. 2 (1988): 1–9.

9. The Diabetes Control and Complications Trial Research Group. "The Effect of Intensive Treatment of Diabetes on the Development and Progression of Long-Term Complications in Insulin-Dependent Diabetes Mellitus." *New England Journal of Medicine* 329, no. 14 (1993): 977–86.

10. American Diabetes Association. "The Pharmacologic Treatment of Hyperglycemia in NIDDM." *Diabetes Care* 18, no. 11 (1995): 1,510–18.

11. Pyorala, K. "Relationship of Glucose Tolerance and Plasma Insulin to the Incidence of Coronary Heart Dis-

ease: Results from Two Population Studies in Finland." *Diabetes Care* 2 (1979): 131–41.

12. Fontbonne, A., et al. "Hyperinsulinemia as a Predictor of Coronary Heart Disease Mortality in a Healthy Population: The Paris Prospective Study, 15-year follow-up." *Diabetologia* 34 (1991): 356–61.

13. Ducimetiere, P., et al. "Relationship of Plasma Insulin Levels to the Incidence of Myocardial Infarction and Coronary Heart Disease Mortality in a Middle-Aged Population." *Diabetologia* 19 (1980): 205–10.

14. Despres, J.P., et al. "Hyperinsulinemia as an Independent Risk Factor for Ischemic Heart Disease (The Quebec Cardiovascular Study)." *New England Journal of Medicine* 334, no. 15 (1996): 952–57.

15. Kuusisto, J., et al. "Hyperinsulinemic microalbuminuria: A New Risk Indicator for Coronary Heart Disease." *Circulation* 91, no. 3 (1995): 831–37.

16. Ferrara, A., Barrett-Conner, E.L., and Edelstein, S.L. "Hyperinsulinemia Does Not Increase the Risk of Fatal Cardiovascular Disease in Elderly Men or Women without Diabetes: The Rancho Bernardo Study." *American Journal of Epidemiology* 140, no.10 (1994): 857–69.

17. Mazze, R.S., et al. "Staged Diabetes Management: Toward an Integrated Model of Diabetes Care." *Diabetes Care* 17, suppl 1 (1994): 56–66.

18. Ohkubo, Y. et al. "Intensive Insulin Therapy Prevents the Progression of Diabetic Microvascular Complications in Japanese Patients with Non-insulin-dependent Diabetes Mellitus: A Randomized Prospective 6-year Study." *Diabetes Research and Clinical Practice* 28 (1995): 103–17.

19. Knatterud, G.L., et al. "Effects of Hypoglycemic Agents on Vascular Complications in Patients with Adult-Onset Diabetes VII. Mortality and Selected Nonfatal Events with Insulin Treatment." *Journal of American Medical Association* 240, no. 1 (1978): 37–42.

20. United Kingdom Prospective Diabetes Study Group. "Overview of 6 Years' Therapy of Type II Diabetes: A Progressive Disease (UKPDS)." *Diabetes* 44 (1995): 1,249–58.

21. Turner, R., Cull, D., and Holman, R., for the UKPDS study group. "United Kingdom Prospective Diabetes Study 17: A 9-Year Update of a Randomized, Controlled Trial of the Effect of Improved Metabolic Control on Complications in Non–Insulin-Dependent Diabetes Mellitus." *Annals of Internal Medicine* 124, no. 1 pt 2 (1996): 136–45.

22. Gerich, J.E. "Oral Hypoglycemic Agents." *New England Journal of Medicine* 321, no.18 (1989): 1,231–45.

23. Calle-Pascual, A.L., et al. "Comparison between Acarbose, Metformin, and Insulin Treatment in Type 2 Diabetic Patients with Secondary Failure to Sulfonylurea Treatment." *Diabete et Metabolisme* 21, no. 4 (1995): 256–60.

24. Bailey, C.J. "Biguanides and NIDDM." *Diabetes Care* 15, no. 6 (1992): 755–72.

25. Giugliano, D., et al. "Metformin Improves Glucose, Lipid Metabolism, and Reduces Blood Pressure in Hypertensive, Obese Women." *Diabetes Care* 16, no.10 (1993): 1,387–90.

26. Bailey, C.J. and Turner, R.C. "Metformin." *New England Journal of Medicine* 334, no.9 (1996): 574–79.

27. Coniff, R.F., Shapiro, J.A., and Seaton, T.B. "Long-Term Efficacy and Safety of Acarbose in the Treatment of Obese Subjects with Non–Insulin-Dependent Diabetes Mellitus." *Archives of Internal Medicine* 154 (1994): 2,442–48.

28. Coniff, R.F., et al. "Multicenter, Placebo-Controlled Trial Comparing Acarbose with Placebo, Tolbutamide, and Tolbutamide-Plus-Acarbose in Non–Insulin-Dependent Diabetes Mellitus." *The American Journal of Medicine* 98 (1995): 443–51.

29. Balfour, J.A. and McTavish, D. "Acarbose. An Update of its Pharmacology and Therapeutic Use in Diabetes Mellitus." *Drugs* 46, no. 6 (1993): 1,025–54.

30. Vannasaeng, S., et al. "Effects of Alpha-Glucosidase Inhibitor (Acarbose) Combined with Sulfonylurea or Sulfonylurea and Metformin in Treatment of Non–Insulin-Dependent Diabetes Mellitus." *Journal of the Medical Association of Thailand* 78, no.11 (1995): 578–85.

31. Simcic, K.J., et al. "Crossover Comparison of Maximum Dose Glyburide and Glipizide." *Southern Medical Journal* 84, no.6 (1991): 743–46.

32. Berelowitz, M., et al. "Comparative Efficacy of a Once-Daily Controlled-Release Formulation of Glipizide and Immediate-Release Glipizide in Patients with NIDDM." *Diabetes Care* 17, no. 12 (1994): 1,460–64.

33. Groop, L.C., et al. "Hyperglycemia and Absorption of Sulfonylurea Drugs." *Lancet* July 15 (1989): 129–30.

34. DeFronzo, R.A., Goodman, A.M., and the Multicenter Metformin Study Group. "Efficacy of Metformin in Patients with Non–Insulin-Dependent Diabetes Mellitus." *New England Journal of Medicine* 333, no. 9 (1995): 541–49.

35. Bayraktar, M., Van Thiel, D.H., and Adalar, N. "A Comparison of Acarbose Versus Metformin as an Adjuvant Therapy in Sulfonylurea-Treated NIDDM Patients." *Diabetes Care* 19, no. 3 (1996): 252–54.

36. Chiasson, J.L., et al. "The Efficacy of Acarbose in the Treatment of Patients with Non–Insulin-Dependent Diabetes Mellitus." *Annals of Internal Medicine* 121, no.12 (1994): 928–35.

37. Johnson, J.L., Wolf, S.L., and Kabadi, U.M. "Efficacy of Insulin and Sulfonylurea Combination Therapy in Type II Diabetes: A Meta-Analysis of the Randomized Placebo-Controlled Trials." *Archives of Internal Medicine* 156 (1996): 259–64.

38. Giugliano, D., et al. "Metformin for Obese, Insulin-Treated Diabetic Patients: Improvement in Glycemic Control and Reduction of Metabolic Risk Factors." *European Journal of Clinical Pharmacology* 44 (1993): 107–12.

39. White, J.R. "The Pharmacologic Management of Patients with Type II Diabetes Mellitus in the Era of New Oral Agents and Insulin Analogs." *Diabetes Spectrum* 9, no. 4 (1996): 227–34.

40. Abraira, C., et al. "Veterans Affairs Cooperative Study on Glycemic Control and Complications in Type II Diabetes (VA-CSDM)." *Diabetes Care* 18, no. 8 (1995): 1,113–23.

CHAPTER 2

Important Aspects of Self-Management Education in Patients with Diabetes

Darren M. Stam, PharmD and John P. Graham, PharmD

The Diabetes Control and Complications Trial has shown that the long-term complications of diabetes can be decreased with intensive glycemic control. However, comprehensive patient education is required to provide the patient with the self-management skills necessary to achieve this level of glycemic control. Epidemiologic data indicate that large numbers of patients do not receive the proper care or education necessary to develop such self-management abilities. In order to convey the importance of patient education, the American Diabetes Association (ADA) has labeled self-management education as a cornerstone of therapy for patients with diabetes. Standards of care have also been defined by the ADA. Within the current U.S. health care system, however, limitations are present that may affect the quality of care and ability to provide adequate patient education. Therefore, it is the responsibility of the health care provider to improve the education process in an attempt to maintain standards of care outlined by the ADA. When developing a diabetes self-management training program, the ADA national standards can be used as a guideline. Key words: *diabetes mellitus, disease state complications, clinical practice guidelines, health care team, lifestyle modifications, patient education, patient outcomes, pharmacologic therapy, self-management training, therapy goals*

INTRODUCTION

Diabetes mellitus (Type I and Type II) is a chronic metabolic illness that affects approximately 5 percent of the U.S. population or about 16 million people.[1,2] Prolonged hyperglycemia in the patient with diabetes can result in both micro- and macrovascular complications that ultimately contribute to the morbidity and mortality associated with the disease.[3–6] The Diabetes Control and Complications Trial (DCCT) concluded, however, that with intensive glucose control the incidence of long-term microvascular complications such as retinopathy, nephropathy, and neuropathy could be reduced as much as 50 percent–70 percent when compared to more conventional therapy.[7] The DCCT patient popu-

lation consisted of patients with Type I diabetes, and to date, there has not been a trial such as this one that included patients with Type II diabetes. It has been postulated, however, that similar mechanisms are responsible for the development of such complications in those with Type II diabetes and that intensive therapy would most likely have similar benefits in this patient population as well.[5]

Since the publication of the DCCT, the American Diabetes Association (ADA) has promoted "tighter" treatment goals through their Clinical Practice Guidelines.[8,9] As physicians and other health care providers become more aware of these guidelines, it is likely that there will be a greater attempt to comply with these more intensive goals of therapy when treating diabetes in hopes of preventing or delaying the progression of long-term complications.

Tight control, however, is not achieved without extra work. Implications of the DCCT show that such intensive treatment requires comprehensive training and patient education in the self-management of the disease.[7,8,10,11] And, indeed, many studies have shown that diabetes patient education clearly has a beneficial effect with regard to desirable outcomes such as improved knowledge and self-care behaviors, better metabolic control, and reduced complications.[12,13] Unfortunately, large numbers of the diabetes patient population do not receive the proper care or education necessary to adequately achieve and maintain intensive glycemic control.[14-17]

Epidemiologic data from the National Health Interview Survey (NHIS) show that approximately 10 percent of patients with diabetes, Type I and Type II included, do not have a physician for the regular care of their diabetes and 32 percent of those with a physician had fewer than four office visits each year.[14-18] Most of these visits were not made to a diabetes specialist, but rather to their usual primary care physician. Likewise, only about 35 percent of individuals with diabetes have attended a diabetes class or education program and only about 33 percent check their blood sugars on a regular basis.[14,15,18,19]

In an attempt to improve diabetes care, and hopefully overcome the current lack of education in the diabetes patient population, the ADA has recognized the importance of promoting patient education and has labeled self-management training as a "cornerstone of treatment for all people with diabetes."[20(p.5114)] Objectives for diabetes education have also been identified and include the following[20,21]:

- improving the patients' knowledge and skills with respect to their disease
- promoting positive behavior changes
- improving patient outcomes by decreasing complications and hospitalizations while improving the patients' overall quality of life

In essence, we want patients to attain the appropriate knowledge, skills, and attitudes necessary to self-manage their disease. Taking this one step further, pharmacists and other health care professionals should focus on four general areas when educating patients with diabetes. These aspects include the following:

1. adequate understanding of the disease state and potential complications
2. expected goals of therapy and importance of self-management
3. awareness of lifestyle modifications and risk factor reduction
4. understanding of the medical regimen and how to monitor therapy

Appropriate education should ensure that patients walk away with a firm understanding of these areas and the ability to use the knowledge and skills obtained to self-manage their disease. A guideline on counseling the patient with diabetes regarding these particular aspects of patient education is outlined below.

ASPECTS OF PATIENT EDUCATION

Understanding of Disease State and Complications

Disease State

In order for diabetic patients to ultimately obtain the ability to self-manage their disease, they must first obtain an adequate understanding of the disease state itself. Many patients remain in the dark about what is going on with their bodies and why their blood sugars are elevated. In the past, the health care system has typically perceived diabetes as a "mild illness" due to the relatively asymptomatic nature of the disease and the latency period between the onset of hyperglycemia and long-term complications.[16,17] This is particularly so in patients with Type II diabetes who comprise the majority of the overall diabetes population. Patients were often not told of the potential complications that could occur if blood sugars remained uncontrolled and how these complications could be prevented or delayed with adequate glucose control. Without goals and expectations, motivation in treating the disease by the physician and the patient is inadequate and obviously not an appropriate setting for the intensive treatment of diabetes.

In order to change these misconceptions about diabetes, patients need to begin with an adequate understanding of the disease state and complications, both acute and chronic, that can occur as a result of uncontrolled hyperglycemia. An understanding of the seriousness of the disease may spark the motivation necessary for patients to become active in their disease management. Newly diagnosed diabetics should first be introduced to the "normal" levels of blood sugar (Table 1) and how their current blood glucose control compares to these levels. A simple explanation should be given as to why their sugars are elevated while incorporating a brief and simple summary of the pathogenesis of the disease while being specific for Type I or Type II patients. Using a figure or illustration that depicts the pathogenesis of the disease may help patients visualize and better understand what is going wrong.

Acute Complications

Acute complications that can potentially occur in those with diabetes are symptomatic hyper- and/or hypoglycemia, diabetic ketoacidosis (DKA), hyperglycemic hyperosmolar nonketotic syndrome (HHNS), and an increased risk to acquire infections. All patients with diabetes should be taught to recognize these problems along with factors that predispose to them. Subsequently, patients should learn to assess and manage these complications appropriately.

Hyper- and hypoglycemia are probably the most common complications that both Type I and Type II patients may face. Recognizing the fact that one has symptomatic hyperglycemia may trigger the patient to seek medical care sooner or to evaluate his or her own therapy to determine what may be going wrong and/or what changes need to be made. Also, since more intensive glucose control has been shown to lead to a significantly greater incidence of hypoglycemic episodes,[7] then the patient's ability to recognize this problem and take action, if and when it occurs, is very important. To develop this ability, patients should be able to recognize the signs and symptoms of hyper- and hypoglycemia, potential causes for these problems, and ultimately, how to manage them (see the box, "Signs, Symptoms, and Management of Hyper/Hypoglycemia").[22,23] Friends and family members should also be educated on the management of hypoglycemia, especially with regard to the use of glucagon for situations in which the patient is unconscious or unable to take food by mouth.

DKA (more common in Type I diabetes) and HHNS (more common in Type II diabetes) can be severe and life threatening. Acute stressors (e.g., infection, trauma) may predispose patients to DKA or HHNS. Because of this, the concept of sick-day management is important and should be included as part of the overall education process.[24,25] Patients should develop an understanding of what types of situations may adversely affect glucose control and predispose them to DKA or HHNS. The following points should be covered when discussing sick-day management: (1) pa-

Table 1. Goals of therapy based on the ADA guidelines

Monitoring parameter	Normal	Goal	Action suggested
Preprandial glucose (mg/dL)	<115	80–120	<80 or >140
Postprandial glucose (mg/dL)	<140	<180	>180
Bedtime glucose (mg/dL)	<120	100–140	<100 or >160
Hemoglobin A$_{1c}$ (%)*	<6%	<7%	>8%

*Referenced to a normal range of 4%–6%.
Adapted from *Diabetes Care* 19, Suppl. 1 (1996): S8–S15.

Signs, Symptoms, and Management of Hyper/Hypoglycemia

Hyperglycemia

Signs and symptoms
- Polyuria (frequent urination)
- Polydipsia (excessive thirst)
- Polyphagia (excessive hunger)
- Fatigue, drowsiness
- Weight loss—primarily in Type I patients
- Blurred vision
- Dry skin
- Nausea
- Frequent infections (e.g., vaginal, urinary tract infections)
- Diabetic ketoacidosis—ketonuria, fruity odor of acetone on breath

Possible causes
- Acute stress (e.g., infection, trauma, surgery, psychological)
- Dehydration
- Decreased physical activity
- Poor dietary habits (overeating)
- Menstruation
- Inactive insulin (e.g., improper storage, outdated or crystallized insulin)
- Other drugs (e.g., beta-blockers, diuretics, glucocorticoids, niacin, sympathomimetics)

Treatment
- Determine and correct underlying cause
- Anticipate need for changes in therapeutic regimen or more frequent physician follow-up

Hypoglycemia

Signs and symptoms
- Nausea
- Dizziness/lightheadedness
- Blurred vision
- Cold sweats, sweaty palms
- Hunger
- Confusion, anxiety, irritability
- Nightmares, restless sleep
- Morning headaches
- Weakness, fatigue
- Shakiness, rapid heart rate

Possible causes
- Increased exercise
- Irregular eating patterns
- Delayed gastric emptying (gastroparesis)
- Excessive hypoglycemic agents
- Other drugs (e.g., ethanol, anabolic steroids, ACE-inhibitors, sulfonamide antibiotics)

Treatment
- 10–20 gm of carbohydrate (e.g., ½ cup orange juice, milk, or regular soda; ¼ cup grape juice; 2 tsp. sugar; several pieces of hard candy; or 2 B/D glucose tablets)
- If unconscious—Glucagon 1 mg SQ, IM, or IV*

*SQ, IM, or IV (subcutaneous, intramuscular, or intravenous).

tients should take their usual doses of insulin regardless of eating habits or nausea and vomiting, (2) they should monitor blood sugars more frequently (approximately every three to four hours), (3) they should try to maintain fluid and caloric intake (½ cup/hr for adults and 50 gm carbohydrates every four hours), (4) patients with Type I diabetes should test their urine for ketones (especially if blood sugars are greater than 240 mg/dL), and (5) they should contact their physician if blood glucose levels remain above 240 mg/dL or urine ketones remain high.[22,24]

Due to the decreased immune response in the individual with diabetes and the fact that elevated glucose levels provide a superb environment for the growth of microorganisms, common infections can be more prevalent in this patient population. Recurrent infections such as vaginitis, balanitis, and urinary tract infections may be observed. The patient should be aware of this possibility and seek appropriate medical care if these infections occur.

Recognizing acute complications such as these and developing the ability to effectively manage them is one step in the process of patients becoming more proactive in the management of their disease.

Long-term Complications

Diabetes is the leading cause of blindness in those less than 65 years old, the most common cause of renal failure, and a major contributing factor in foot and leg amputations annually.[2,24,26,27] Overt microvascular complications such as retinopathy, nephropathy, and neuropathy may not be detected until many years after the onset of hyperglycemia, but when they occur, they can contribute to significant morbidity and mortality in this patient population.

Patients should be aware of these potential long-term complications and the reasons for their occurrence (e.g., chronically elevated blood sugars, genetic predisposition). Patients should also be advised that these microvascular complications can be delayed or even prevented if blood sugars are adequately controlled. A brief summary of the DCCT results may be worthwhile in certain patients with Type I diabetes, especially in those who have a history of noncompliance or those with poor motivation to control their disease. Macrovascular complications (cardiovascular, peripheral vascular, and/or cerebrovascular disease) may also result from diabetes, especially in patients with other multiple risk factors.[28,29] An understanding of these factors and how they interrelate may also help motivate patients to take responsibility for the self-management of their disease.

Goals of Therapy and Importance of Self-Management

Goals of Therapy

Once patients have a firm understanding of their disease state, they should be introduced to the proposed goals of therapy that have been outlined by the ADA Clinical Practice Guidelines (Table 1).[8] A brief description of the different monitoring parameters should first be given to the patient (i.e., preprandial, postprandial, and bedtime glucose measurements, and hemoglobin A_{1c}), as well as what each value reflects in terms of blood glucose control. They should learn to differentiate between normal values, expected goals of therapy, and values out of range that may necessitate a change in their current therapy or management skills.

The box, "Signs, Symptoms, and Management of Hyper/Hypoglycemia" may provide assistance to patients in determining what their current status is in terms of glucose control, as well as when action should be taken. The patients should also be able to correlate "higher" levels with the increased chance for symptomatic hyperglycemia and complications. Likewise, they should realize that "lower" levels may coincide with increased episodes of hypoglycemia. This step in the overall education of the patient is essential because without an understanding of the goals, the patient will not be able to develop the expectations necessary to take an active role in the management of his or her disease.

Patient Limitations

It has been recognized that aggressive management requires individualization of therapy because intensive glycemic control is inappropriate in certain situations. Therefore, it is important for the health care provider to help patients identify limitations that may impact their ability to achieve intensive therapy goals. Financial or time management problems, unwillingness or inability to actively participate in self-management, persistent symptomatic hypoglycemia, patients in whom hypoglycemia may be dangerous (e.g., elderly, children), or other medical factors that may limit life expectancy are some limitations that may preclude the intensive treatment of diabetes.[11] Alternative goals should be discussed and agreed upon in these situations. It is important that patient input always be considered in the decision-making process to promote the concept of self-management.

Self-Management

After goals of therapy have been discussed and identified and patients have developed an understanding of these goals, it is important to encourage them to take an active role in managing their disease. The importance of self-management in achieving a set of particular goals should be emphasized. Hopefully, patients knowledgeable of the goals of therapy who develop appropriate self-management skills can then begin to develop expectations for their role in the therapeutic regimen. Subsequently, they should learn to compare their treatment outcomes to the standard goals of therapy and determine when action should be taken with regard to the management of their disease.

Nonpharmacologic Therapy and Risk Factor Reduction

Lifestyle modifications are almost always the first line of therapy in patients with diabetes. These measures include diet, exercise, risk factor reduction, preventive therapies, and behavioral modifications. Diet and exercise should always be reinforced as cornerstones of therapy; however, health care professionals may not place enough emphasis on the importance of these measures.

Patients need to be told why these modes of therapy are important and how they can help to improve control of the disease. Successful diet and exercise therapy, although less important in Type I diabetes, will help promote weight loss, which can improve the body's ability to utilize insulin and improve the lipid profile. Also, benefits with regard to improved glucose control and blood pressure reduction have been shown even with weight reductions of as little as 10–20 pounds (5–10 kg).[30] Optimizing these modes of therapy may lengthen the time before pharmacologic agents are necessary.

Diet

Currently, there is no specific diet to be followed by the diabetic individual. Although we have heard of "ADA" or "diabetic" diets in the past, today's dietary plan is based on nutritional assessment and treatment goals.[30] Nutrition therapy should be individualized, considering factors such as usual eating habits, current glycemic control, personal lifestyle, and diabetes management goals. It is important that any patients taking insulin develop a regular eating and exercise schedule that is consistent with the onset of action and duration of the insulin preparation used. Nutritional therapy for the patient with Type II diabetes should help achieve glucose, lipid, and blood pressure control.[30]

The use of artificial sweeteners is acceptable in individuals with diabetes. Also, the ADA does not prohibit the consumption of alcoholic beverages by patients with diabetes, when used in moderation. However, the caloric contribution and potential hypoglycemic effect of alcohol should be considered.[30] For further information regarding diet therapy, the reader is referred elsewhere.[30-33] A registered dietician, who can provide the necessary recommendations for appropriate nutritional therapy, should be consulted.

Exercise

Before beginning an exercise program, patients should be evaluated by their physician to identify problems that may preclude certain types of exercise regimens.[34] After physician screening has taken place and exercise modalities have been discussed, patients should be counseled on strategies for the incorporation of exercise into their overall self-management plan. In doing so, patients should become aware of several important points.

First of all, it is important that patients be taught to test blood sugars before and after exercise, especially in those with Type I diabetes. Patients taking insulin will be more susceptible to episodes of hypoglycemia than patients on oral agents. Therefore, patients should carefully plan the exercise regimen around dietary and insulin schedules.[34,35] Exercise should be avoided or delayed if fasting blood sugars are greater than 250–300 mg/dL, especially in the presence of a positive urine ketone test. If blood glucose levels are less that 80–100 mg/dL before exercise, extra carbohydrates should be ingested.[35]

Second, patients should be encouraged to learn and anticipate the glycemic response for a particular type of exercise and keep extra carbohydrate-containing foods available during and after exercise for cases of hypoglycemia. These points are more important for those individuals with Type I diabetes. In addition, exercise may increase subcutaneous blood flow and increase the rate of insulin absorption. To minimize increases in the absorption of regular insulin during exercise, the patient should be advised to avoid injections of insulin in areas of working muscle or delay exercise for approximately 30 minutes to an hour after an injection.[35] All patients should continue to monitor for signs and symptoms of hypoglycemia (see the box, "Signs, Symptoms, and Management of Hyper/Hypoglycemia") after exercise.

Risk Factor Reduction

With the increased incidence of macrovascular complications among patients with diabetes, eliminating or reducing risk factors that may predispose one to these complications is an important aspect of overall therapy.[28,29] At every counseling session, the health care provider should reinforce the importance of eliminating or controlling risk factors when they are present. Several of these include smoking cessation, control of hypertension and dyslipidemias, moderation of alcohol intake, and weight reduction.

Preventive Measures

Certain preventive measures should be included in the education of diabetic individuals in an attempt to identify and possibly eliminate problems before they occur. With appropriate foot hygiene, the risk of development of diabetes foot infections that could potentially lead to hospitalization and amputation can be reduced or even prevented.[27,36] Appropriate foot care is one aspect of preventive care that patients with diabetes can conduct themselves or with the assistance of a friend or family member.

Education must ensure that the patient understand the reasons for proper foot care. This should include a brief explanation of the relationships between neuropathic and/or vascular complications and the occurrence of foot problems.[36] All patients should be educated on appropriate foot hygiene, avoidance of foot trauma, proper footwear, and what to do if problems develop.[36, 37] The box, "General Foot Care Guidelines," contains some general guidelines on appropriate foot care. The individual with diabetes should also be reminded of the importance of annual ophthalmologic exams, proper dental hygiene, and occasional monitoring for urine protein.

General Foot Care Guidelines

Suggestions for Proper Foot Hygiene

- Inspect feet daily for minor trauma (blisters, cuts, etc.); use mirror for bottom of feet.
- Cut toenails straight across and buff calluses.
- Do not perform "bathroom surgery" on foot problems; see a physician or podiatrist instead.
- Avoid using "over-the-counter" preparations to treat foot problems such as corns or calluses.
- Wash feet in water that is not too hot or cold and avoid soaking; dry feet carefully.
- Avoid walking barefoot, especially on hot or rough surfaces.
- Wear socks and shoes that fit well; inspect for deformities that may cause abnormal rubbing.
- Avoid sandals with thongs and do not wear shoes without socks.
- During winter, wear wool socks and protective footwear.
- Avoid crossing legs while sitting as this can place pressure on blood vessels and nerves.
- Ask for help from a friend or family member if eyesight is poor or range of motion is limited.

Team Approach

A multidisciplinary team approach is the best setting for optimizing patient education in diabetes.[8] A health care team that includes a certified diabetes educator, dietitian, podiatrist, ophthalmologist, physician, and pharmacist can provide appropriate patient education specific for each respective area of practice. However, all educators should try to reinforce the different aspects of lifestyle modifications, risk factor reduction, and nonpharmacologic therapy when possible, to ensure adequate patient understanding and compliance.

Pharmacologic Therapy and Monitoring

Education regarding pharmacologic therapy can encompass a large amount of information, especially with the new additions to the pharmacologic armamentarium. In order to minimize toxicities and enhance effectiveness, pharmacologic therapy requires close medical supervision and continuous patient education and follow-up. An adequate understanding of how the drug(s) works, proper administration, potential adverse effects, and monitoring are all important points that should be reviewed with the patient. Although detailed explanations of all available agents is beyond the scope of this article, aspects important in education will be covered.

Hypoglycemic Agents

Sulfonylureas and insulin have been the mainstay of pharmacologic therapy in diabetes for many years. The main adverse effect of these agents is hypoglycemia. Insulin replaces low or nonexistent endogenous insulin in Type I diabetes or insulin-requiring Type II diabetes patients, and sulfonylureas act by stimulating insulin production and/or increasing insulin sensitivity in those with a functioning pancreas (Type II diabetes patients). Both of these agents lower glucose levels, even in the nondiabetic individual, hence they are labeled "hypoglycemic agents." One of the most important aspects in educating patients is establishing an awareness of the hypoglycemic potential of these agents and the importance of home blood glucose monitoring in screening for such reactions. Patients on insulin should have an adequate understanding of the type of insulin they are taking, the onset and duration of action of their preparation(s), instruction with regard to appropriate mixing procedures, injection technique, and storage (see the box, "Insulin Administration").[38]

Antihyperglycemic Agents

Metformin (Glucophage®) and acarbose (Precose®) are two new agents used in the treatment of diabetes. Both of these drugs are accurately described as antihyperglycemic agents because although they lower blood glucose levels, they do not cause hypoglycemia in those who do not have diabetes. In contrast to the sulfonylureas, these agents do not stimulate insulin secretion.

With regard to metformin, probably the most important aspect of patient education involves its potential to cause lactic acidosis. Although rare (~1/33,000 per year), lactic acidosis can be fatal in up to 50 percent of cases.[39,40] Therefore, it is critical for patients to be aware of this potential side effect, have an understanding of what lactic acidosis actually is, and be able to recognize the signs and symptoms of lactic acidosis and predisposing factors for its occurrence. Patients should be reassured that the risk of developing lactic acidosis is low as long as their liver and kidneys are functioning properly, as these help remove the lactic acid from the body to prevent its accumulation. Other predisposing factors include excessive alcohol use (chronic and acute "binge drinking"); severe dehydration; certain X-ray procedures when injectable contrast dyes are used; surgery; or acute complications such as a heart attack, severe infection, or stroke.[39,40]

Symptoms of lactic acidosis include excessive fatigue or weakness, unusual muscle pain, trouble breathing (rapid or labored respirations), unusual abdominal discomfort that is different than that observed during initiation of therapy, feeling unusually cold, dizziness or lightheadedness, or the development of an unusually slow or irregular heart rate.[39,40] The patient should be in-

---

Insulin Administration

Dosing facts
- Administer regular insulin 30–60 minutes before meal.
- Administer lispro insulin (Humalog®) about 15 minutes before meal.
- Lispro and regular insulins are equivalent on a unit per unit basis.

Preparation procedure
- Inspect regular insulin for cloudiness or crystallization.
- Mix intermediate or long-acting insulin vial by rolling in hands.
- Wipe top of vial with alcohol swab.
- Inject a volume of air into the vial equal to the amount of insulin to be withdrawn.
- Invert vial and withdraw insulin.
- Remove excess air from syringe.
- When mixing regular and NPH, inject air into NPH vial first and then into regular vial, then withdraw the regular insulin first.
- Be sure there are no air bubbles in the syringe before injection.

Injection technique
- Wipe injection site with alcohol and allow to air dry.
- Do not tense muscles at site of injection area at time of injection.
- Administer SQ* at a 45° to 90° angle.
- Drawing back on the injected syringe to check for blood is not necessary.
- Sites for injection include the upper arm, anterior and lateral aspects of thigh, abdomen (excluding circle with 2-inch radius around navel), and buttocks.
- Rotate injection sites within one area and then switch to another area; rotating sites can help prevent lipodystrophies.
- Do not reuse needles after they become dull.

Storage
- Refrigerate all vials not in use.
- Opened vials being used may be kept at room temperature for approximately 30 days.
- Prefilled syringes are good for up to 3 weeks when stored in a refrigerator; these should be stored in a vertical position with the needles facing upward to avoid suspended insulin particles from clogging the needle.

*Subcutaneous.

---

structed to contact his or her physician or pharmacist if any of these symptoms occur, or if they have any acute illness such as severe vomiting, diarrhea, and/or fever, or if fluid intake is significantly reduced. Patients should inform their physicians that they are taking metformin when surgery or X-rays with injectable contrast dye is planned. If any of these situations occur, metformin may have to be held temporarily. The importance of alcohol restriction should be emphasized with all patients.

Other side effects with metformin are minor and transient and usually occur in the first few weeks of therapy but decrease with time. These include diarrhea, metallic taste, and nausea and stomach upset.[39,40] Taking the agent with meals can help to reduce these side effects. Also, starting with lower doses such as 500 mg once or twice daily may also minimize the severity of these initial gastrointestinal complaints.[39,40]

Acarbose reduces the postprandial rise in glucose by delaying the digestion and absorption of sugars, starches, and complex carbohydrates.[41,42] Due to its mechanism of action, there are several limiting side effects that patients should know. Gastrointestinal effects such as flatulence, abdominal bloating, and diarrhea occur frequently in up to 80 percent of those taking the drug.[41,42] These events are not always transient in nature as they are with metformin.

Dosing should be titrated to minimize these adverse events. The initial starting dose was 25 mg (one half of a 50 mg tablet) three times a day with the first bite of each meal; however, new recommendations suggest starting at 25 mg daily and increasing the dose slowly in order to further minimize gastrointestinal complaints.[41,42] These side effects may also be minimized by avoiding dietary sources of sucrose as this may potentiate gastrointestinal complaints. Titration should be slow (every four to eight weeks) and be based on one-hour postprandial blood glucose readings. Patients should be instructed to check both fasting and one-hour postprandial glucose levels.

Although acarbose alone should not cause hypoglycemia, it is important to educate patients about how to manage hypoglycemia if they are also taking a sulfonylurea or insulin in combination. Glucose tablets or gel must be utilized since the absorption of sugar from candy or other complex carbohydrates may be delayed in the presence of acarbose. Skim milk may also be used.

Self-Monitoring

Home blood glucose monitoring is an important aspect in the overall self-management plan of patients with diabetes. Only a small percentage of these patients self-monitor their blood glucose levels.[14,19] It is important that patients receive the appropriate education and training to enforce the importance of blood glucose monitoring.

Self-monitoring of blood glucose can help assist patients and health care providers in several areas.[43] These include providing patients with the means by which they can achieve and maintain a specific set of glycemic goals, prevent and/or detect hypoglycemia, avoid prolonged hyperglycemia, and adjust therapy in response to changes that may adversely affect blood glucose levels (e.g., acute illness, exercise, diet changes, other medications).[43] If patients realize the importance of home blood glucose monitoring and actively engage in self-management, they can use the results of their tests to self-adjust diet, exercise or medical therapy; identify and properly manage hyper- and hypoglycemia; and improve decision-making and problem-solving abilities.[43]

Readings should be recorded in log books or in the memory of specific home-monitoring devices. Documenting the time of the reading with respect to meals, exercise, and medication dosing is also important for appropriate interpretation by the patient and health care personnel. Patients must be educated with regard to the proper use of their particular monitoring device and, subsequently, learn to integrate the data obtained to help achieve the ability to self-manage their disease. The effective use of home blood glucose monitors will encourage patients to assume a greater responsibility for control and enforce the concept of self-management.[43] Urine glucose monitoring can be considered when patients are unable or unwilling to perform blood glucose testing.[8,43]

•   •   •

To achieve and maintain near-normal glycemia, similar to that attained by the intensive treatment group in the DCCT, close and frequent follow-up by a multifaceted health care team is necessary. Patients also must have the knowledge, skills, and attitudes necessary to assume an active role in their disease self-management.[7,8] Current practice in the U.S. health care system, however, often does not provide the setting necessary for such intensive care. Results from the NHIS support this fact.[14] These current trends do not provide the comprehensive follow-up and education necessary for the intensive management of the diabetes patient population.[16–18]

Changes needed in the current U.S. health care system to promote improved care for patients with diabetes have been identified; however, barriers still exist that limit the quality of care that is necessary to achieve the control needed to decrease complications.[16,17] Some of these proposed changes would require a significant amount of restructuring within the current health care system. However, the fact remains that patient education has resulted in positive outcomes, including increased rates of blood glucose monitoring, compliance with overall management, improved glucose control, and reduced incidence of complications.[12,13,19] Therefore, it has been recommended that health care providers begin to develop programs, both individually and collaboratively, to improve the patient education process.[15,20,44,45] The fundamental role of patient education in those with diabetes has been addressed and defined in the standards of care set forth by the ADA.[8,20] These standards can be used as a guide for the establishment and maintenance of quality diabetes patient education or self-management education programs.[8,20]

Pharmacists are in an ideal position to interact with patients and provide the necessary educa-

tion to improve self-management abilities in those with diabetes. We, then, are helping to achieve the standards of care outlined by the ADA. It is also our responsibility to increase patient and public awareness of the seriousness of diabetes and the importance of appropriate management. To provide this essential service may necessitate that some health care personnel obtain additional training in the current theories and standards of diabetes care.

REFERENCES

1. CDC. "National Diabetes Awareness Month." *Morbidity and Mortality Weekly Report* 45, no. 43 (1996).

2. American Diabetes Association. *Diabetes 1993 Vital Statistics.* Alexandria, VA: ADA, 1993.

3. Nathan, D.M. "The Pathophysiology of Diabetic Complications: How Much Does the Glucose Hypothesis Explain?" *Annals of Internal Medicine* 124, no. 1, pt.2 (1996): 86–89.

4. Genuth, S.M. "The Case for Blood Glucose Control." *Advances in Internal Medicine* 40 (1995): 573–623.

5. Klein, R., Klein, D.E.K., and Moss, D.E. "Relation of Glycemic Control to Diabetic Microvascular Complications in Diabetes Mellitus." *Annals of Internal Medicine* 124, no. 1, pt.2 (1996): 90–96.

6. Klein, R. "Hyperglycemia and Microvascular and Macrovascular Disease in Diabetes." *Diabetes Care* 18, no. 2 (1995): 258–68.

7. The Diabetes Control and Complications Trial Research Group. "The Effect of Intensive Treatment of Diabetes on the Development and Progression of Long-Term Complications in Insulin-Dependent Diabetes Mellitus." *New England Journal of Medicine* 329, no. 14 (1993): 977–86.

8. American Diabetes Association. "Standards of Medical Care for Patients with Diabetes Mellitus (Position Statement)." *Diabetes Care* 19, Suppl. 1 (1996): S8–S15.

9. American Diabetes Association. "Standards of Medical Care for Patients with Diabetes Mellitus (Position Statement)." *Diabetes Care* 17 (1994): 616–23.

10. Harris, M.I., Eastman, R.L., and Siebert, C. "The DCCT and Medical Care for Diabetes in the U.S." *Diabetes Care* 17, no. 7 (1994): 761–64.

11. Henry, R.R., and Genuth, S. "Forum One: Current Recommendations about Intensification of Metabolic Control in Non–Insulin-Dependent Diabetes Mellitus." *Annals of Internal Medicine* 124, no. 1, pt.2 (1996): 175–77.

12. Brown, S.A. "Studies of Educational Interventions and Outcomes in Diabetic Adults: A Meta-Analysis Revis-

ited." *Patient Education and Counselling* 16 (1990): 189–215.

13. Padgett, D., Mumford, E., Hynes, M., and Carter, K. "Meta-Analysis of the Effects of Educational and Psychosocial Interventions on Management of Diabetes Mellitus." *Journal of Clinical Epidemiology* 40, no. 10 (1988): 1,007–30.

14. Harris, M.I. "Medical Care for Patients with Diabetes—Epidemiologic Aspects." *Annals of Internal Medicine* 124, no. 1, pt.2 (1996): 117–22.

15. Coonrod, B.A., Harris, M.I., and Betschart, J. "Frequency and Determinants of Diabetes Patient Education among Adults in the U.S. Population." *Diabetes Care* 17, no. 8 (1994): 852–58.

16. Hiss, R.G. "Barriers to Care in Non–Insulin-Dependent Diabetes Mellitus—The Michigan Experience." *Annals of Internal Medicine* 124, no. 1, pt.2 (1996): 146–48.

17. Hiss, R.G., and Greenfield, S. "Forum Three: Changes in the U.S. Health Care System That Would Facilitate Improved Care for Non–Insulin-Dependent Diabetes Mellitus." *Annals of Internal Medicine* 124, no. 1, pt.2 (1996): 180–83.

18. Harris, M.I., Eastman, R.C., and Siebert, C. "The DCCT and Medical Care for Diabetes in the U.S." *Diabetes Care* 17, no. 7 (1994): 761–64.

19. Harris, M.I., Cowie, C.C., and Howie, L.J. "Self-Monitoring of Blood Glucose by Adults with Diabetes in the United States Population." *Diabetes Care* 16, no. 8 (1993): 1,116–23.

20. American Diabetes Association. "National Standards for Diabetes Self-Management Education Programs and ADA Review Criteria (Standards and Review Criteria)." *Diabetes Care* 19, Suppl. 1 (1996): S114–S118.

21. Tobin, C.T. "Can a Nationwide Policy for Office-Based Diabetes Education be Replicated in the United States?" *Diabetes Care* 16, no. 11 (1993): 1,526–27.

22. Cryer, P.E., and Gerich, J.E. "Hypoglycemia in Insulin-Dependent Diabetes Mellitus: Insulin Excess and Defective Glucose Counterregulation." In *Diabetes Melli-*

tus: Theory and Practice, edited by H. Rifkin and D. Porte, Jr. 4th ed. New York: Elsevier, 1990.

23. Cryer, P.E., Fisher, J.N., and Shamoon, H. "Hypoglycemia (Technical Review)." *Diabetes Care* 17 (1994): 734–55.

24. Ley, B., and Goldman, D. "Sick-Day Management: Preparing for the Unexpected." *Diabetes Spectrum* 4 (1991): 173–76.

25. Carter Center of Emory University. "Closing the Gap. The Problems of Diabetes Mellitus in the U.S." *Diabetes Care* 8 (1985): 391.

26. Drury, P., and Watkins, P. "Diabetic Renal Disease and its Prevention." *Clinical Endocrinology* 38 (1993): 445.

27. Bild, D.E., et al. "Lower Extremity Amputations in People with Diabetes: Epidemiology and Prevention." *Diabetes Care* 12 (1989): 24–31.

28. Stamler, J., et al. "Diabetes, Other Risk Factors, and 12-Year Cardiovascular Mortality for Men Screened in the Multiple Risk Factor Intervention Trial." *Diabetes Care* 16, no. 2 (1993): 434–44.

29. American Diabetes Association. "Role of Cardiovascular Risk Factors in Prevention and Treatment of Macrovascular Disease in Diabetes." *Diabetes Care* 16 (1993): 72.

30. American Diabetes Association. "Nutrition Recommendations and Principles for People with Diabetes Mellitus (Position Statement)." *Diabetes Care* 19, Suppl. 1 (1996): S16–S19.

31. Expert Panel on Detection, Evaluation, and Treatment of High Blood Cholesterol in Adults. "Summary of the Second Report of the National Cholesterol Education Program (NCEP) Expert Panel on Detection, Evaluation, and Treatment of High Blood Cholesterol in Adults (Adult Treatment Panel II)." *Journal of the American Medical Association* 269 (1993): 3,015–23.

32. U.S. Department of Agriculture, U.S. Department of Health and Human Services. *Nutrition and Your Health: Dietary Guidelines for Americans.* 3rd ed. Hyattsville, MD: USDA's Human Nutrition Information Service, 1990.

33. U.S. Department of Agriculture. *The Food Guide Pyramid.* Hyattsville, MD: USDA's Human Nutrition Information Service, 1992.

34. American Diabetes Association. "Diabetes Mellitus and Exercise (Position Statement)." *Diabetes Care* 19, Suppl. 1. (1996): S30.

35. Wasserman, D.H., and Zinman, B. "Exercise in Individuals with IDDM (Technical Review)." *Diabetes Care* 17, no. 8 (1994): 924–37.

36. American Diabetes Association. "Foot Care in Patients with Diabetes Mellitus." *Diabetes Care* 19, Suppl. 1 (1996): S23–S24.

37. Fishman, T.D., Freedline, A.D., and Kahn, D. "Putting the Best Foot Forward." *Nursing 96:* 58–60.

38. American Diabetes Association. "Insulin Administration (Position Statement)." *Diabetes Care* 19, Suppl. 1 (1996): S31–S34.

39. Package insert. Glucophage (metformin). Princeton, NJ: Bristol-Myers Squibb Company, 1995.

40. Bailey, C.J., and Turner, R.C. "Metformin (Drug Therapy Review)." *New England Journal of Medicine* 334, no. 9 (1996): 574–79.

41. Package insert. Precose (acarbose). West Haven, CT: Bayer Corporation, Pharmaceutical Division, 1996.

42. Campbell, L.K., White, J.R., and Campbell, R.K. "Acarbose: Its Role in the Treatment of Diabetes Mellitus." *The Annals of Pharmacotherapy* 30, no. 11 (1996): 1,255–62.

43. American Diabetes Association. "Self-Monitoring of Blood Glucose (Consensus Statement)." *Diabetes Care* 19, Suppl. 1 (1996): S62–S66.

44. National Diabetes Advisory Board, National Institutes of Health. *Diabetes Annual Report.* DHHS Pub. No. NIH 93-1587. Washington, DC: U.S. Government Printing Office, 1993.

45. Department of Health and Human Services, Public Health Service. *Healthy People 2000: National Health Promotion and Disease Prevention Objectives.* DHHS Pub. No. PHS 91-50212.Washington, DC: U.S. Government Printing Office, 1991.

CHAPTER 3

Approach to the Treatment of Diabetic Nephropathy

John M. Burke, PharmD, BCPS

Renal failure is a common long-term complication of diabetes mellitus. Stages of diabetic nephropathy have been described that characterize its clinical course. Diabetic nephropathy develops secondary to long-standing hyperglycemia and hemodynamic changes that damage the glomerulus. Therapy that focuses on the control of glomerular pressures and systemic hypertension can slow the progression of proteinuria and deterioration of renal function. Angiotensin converting enzyme (ACE) inhibitors and calcium channel blockers have been demonstrated to be effective in the management of diabetic nephropathy. A systematic approach to the patient with diabetes with annual screening for proteinuria will help identify those individuals early in the course of disease when proper therapy may be most helpful. Key words: *ACE inhibitors, calcium channel blockers, diabetic nephropathy, microalbuminuria, proteinuria, screening*

Long-term complications contribute to significant morbidity and mortality for patients with diabetes mellitus. Diabetic nephropathy accounts for 34.2 percent of patients with end-stage renal disease.[1] Forty percent of patients with Type I diabetes mellitus develop diabetic nephropathy, while only 10 percent–20 percent of patients with Type II diabetes mellitus will develop this complication.[2,3] With over 90 percent of patients having Type II diabetes, however, a greater number of patients develop renal failure from Type II diabetes. Because of the significant impact that diabetic nephropathy has on morbidity and mortality, it is important to implement efforts that prevent or delay renal complications. An understanding of the clinical presentation, pathophysiology, and therapeutic options is important in the development of a systematic approach to the detection and management of diabetic nephropathy.

CLINICAL COURSE

The clinical course of diabetic nephropathy is best described for the patient with Type I diabetes mellitus. Selby et al. described five stages of diabetic nephropathy (Figure 1).[2] At the time of diagnosis of Type I diabetes mellitus, there is evidence of an effect of diabetes on the kidneys. As a consequence of hyperglycemia, glomerular filtration and kidney size are increased (Stage I). Within two to three years of the onset of diabetes, chronic hyperglycemia produces histologic changes in the kidney; the glomerular basement membrane becomes thickened and the mesangium expands (Stage II). Nevertheless, the patient remains clinically asymptomatic. Such histologic changes are not predictive of further progression of diabetic nephropathy. Up to 60 percent of patients with Type I diabetes mellitus will not progress beyond Stage II.

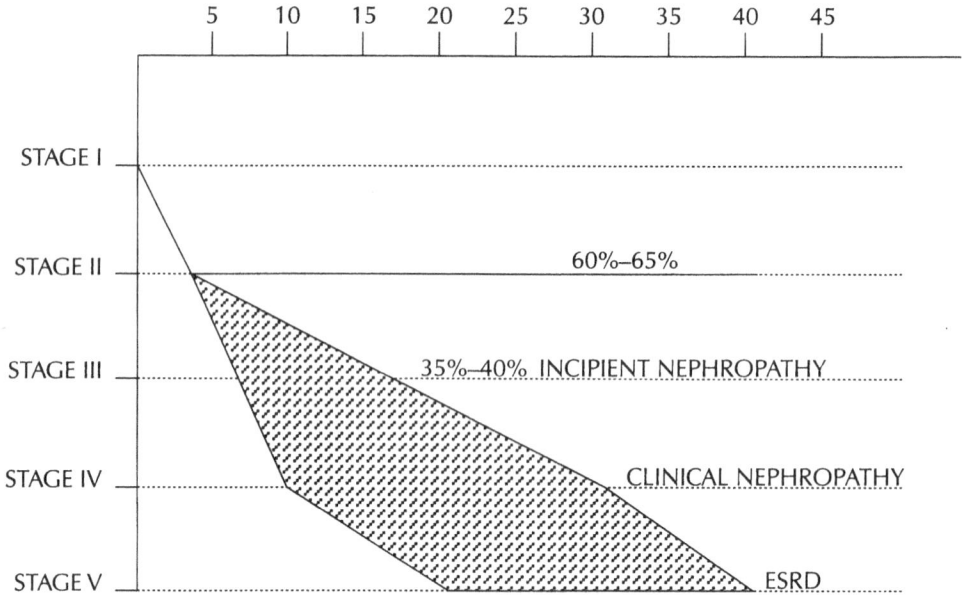

Figure 1. The clinical course of diabetic nephropathy from increased glomerular filtration and kidney size (Stage I) to the development of end-stage renal disease (ESRD) requiring dialysis (Stage V).

Of patients with Type I diabetes mellitus, 35 percent to 40 percent may progress into Stage III within 5–15 years after onset of diabetes.[3] These patients have protein excretion rates of 30–300 mg/day, consisting primarily of albumin. This level of protein excretion (i.e., microalbuminuria) is the earliest manifestation of progressive diabetic nephropathy and is not detectable by standard urinalysis. Over 80 percent of patients in Stage III diabetic nephropathy will experience progressive proteinuria and decline in renal function. Clinically evident diabetic nephropathy with diffuse glomerulosclerosis, overt proteinuria (> 300 mg/day), and declining glomerular filtration marks the onset of Stage IV nephropathy. Renal function often will continue to decline until the patient develops end-stage renal disease requiring dialysis (Stage V). Nelson and the Diabetic Renal Disease Study Group recently described similar progression of nephropathy in patients with Type II diabetes.[4] Early identification of patients and intervention may delay the progression of the disease.

PATHOGENESIS

Because not all patients with diabetes mellitus develop nephropathy, it is postulated that patients are genetically predisposed to the renal complications of hyperglycemia.[3,5,6] For example, African Americans with diabetes mellitus are 3.2–5 times more likely to develop end-stage renal disease than Caucasians.[6] The pathogenesis of diabetic nephropathy is closely related to long-standing hyperglycemia associated with uncontrolled diabetes mellitus (Figure 2). An elevation in blood glucose concentration increases osmotic pressure, which increases afferent arteriolar blood flow and glomerular capillary pressure. An increased responsiveness to the vasoconstrictive effects of angiotensin II also increases glomerular capillary pressure. Increased afferent flow and increased glomerular capillary pressure initially increase glomerular filtration rate (GFR).[3,7] Increased pressure and hyperfiltration change the permeability of glomerular capillaries to proteins, resulting in proteinuria.[3,5,7] Increased

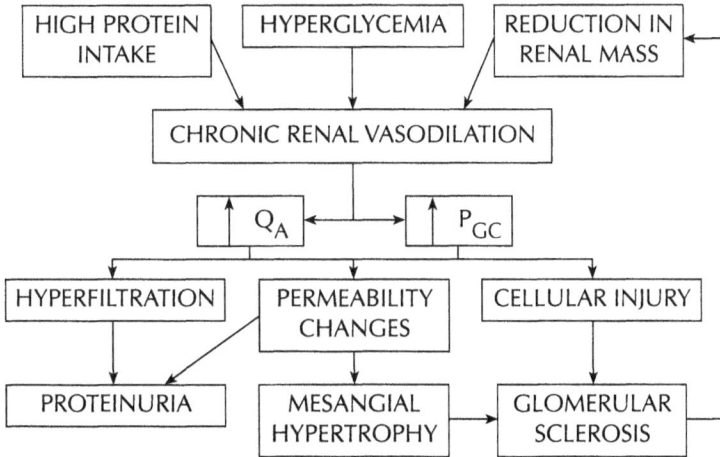

Figure 2. The pathogenesis of diabetic nephropathy.

glomerular pressure and increased flux of protein across capillaries result in mesangial hypertrophy and direct cellular injury, contributing to glomerulosclerosis.[3,7] As the number of functioning nephrons decreases, compensatory afferent arteriolar vasodilatation occurs in the remaining nephrons. This contributes to progressive glomerulosclerosis and renal failure.

Hypertension also contributes to the progression of diabetic nephropathy. Elevated systemic arterial pressure is transmitted through the afferent arteriole and increases glomerular capillary pressure.[3,7] Laffel et al. found that the rate of decline in renal function is proportional to the level of blood pressure in patients with diabetes and proteinuria.[8] An increase in blood pressure, even to high normal values, may contribute to the progression of diabetic nephropathy.

SCREENING

Since the early stages are clinically asymptomatic, a clinical practice that cares for patients with diabetes mellitus must incorporate proper screening. Both qualitative and quantitative tests are available for the detection of urinary protein. Standard urine strips qualitatively detect large amounts of protein (> 150 mg/L). While these

tests are useful in the initial screening, a negative test does not rule out the presence of microalbuminuria. In order to detect microalbuminuria, a random urine collection may be obtained and assessed with either more sensitive strips (such as Micral®) or measurement of the albumin: creatinine ratio. Finally, a timed urine collection can be quantitatively analyzed to determine albumin excretion rate.

The American Diabetes Association (ADA) and the National Kidney Foundation developed a consensus statement regarding diagnosis and treatment of diabetic nephropathy (Figure 3).[9] Because of the latent period prior to the onset of nephropathy, it is recommended that screening be initiated in patients greater than 14 years of age after 5 years from the onset of Type I diabetes.[9] Because the onset of Type II diabetes mellitus can usually not be well established, these patients should be screened at the time of diagnosis. Follow-up screening for each group should be done annually.

The current recommendation is for initial screening with the standard urine strip.[9] If this is negative for protein, a more sensitive strip should be utilized to test for microalbuminuria. If the standard urinalysis is positive, urinary protein excretion should be quantified with a timed

```
        ┌─────────────────────────────┐◄──────────┐
        │  OPTIMIZE GLUCOSE CONTROL   │           │
        └─────────────┬───────────────┘           │
        ┌─────────────▼───────────────┐           │
        │ ANNUAL SCREENING URINE DIPSTICK │        │
        └──┬──────────────────────┬───┘           │
          [+]                    [−]│              │
                        ┌───────────▼──────────┐   │
                        │   MICROALBUMINURIA    │   │
                        │     TEST STRIPS       │   │
                        └────┬──────────────┬───┘   │
                           [+]│           [−]│       │
        ┌───────────────────▼──┐             │       │
        │ 24-HOUR URINE FOR ALBUMIN │        │       │
        │ OR ALBUMIN:CREATININE RATIO │      │       │
        └──┬──────────────────┬─────┘        │       │
          [+]│              [−]│          [NL]│       │
    ┌────────▼──────┐       ┌──▼──────────────▼─┐    │
    │ ACE INHIBITOR │◄──────│     CHECK BP      │    │
    │PROTEIN RESTRICT│ [+HTN]└───────────────────┘   │
    └───────┬───────┘                                │
    ┌───┐   │     NO    ┌──────────────┐  YES  ┌────────┐
    │ADD│◄──┴───────────│  BP < 130/85 │──────►│MONITOR │
    │CCB│               └──────────────┘       └────────┘
    └───┘
```

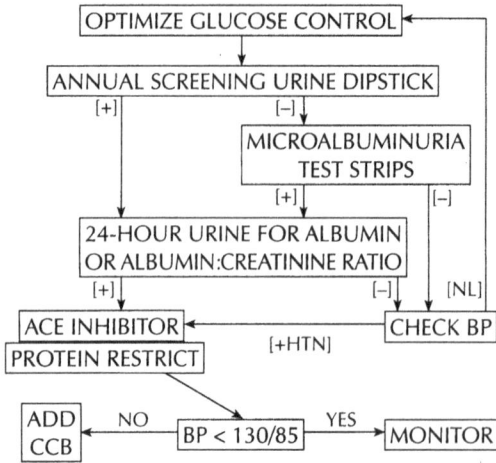

Figure 3. The American Diabetes Association and the National Kidney Foundation's systematic approach to diabetic nephropathy.

urine collection or urine albumin:creatinine ratio to confirm the presence of macroalbuminuria and the need for therapy.[9] If the screen for microalbuminuria is positive, it is recommended that urine albumin excretion be quantified using a timed urine collection.[9] These recommendations should provide a systematic approach to identifying those patients who would benefit from therapy.

MANAGEMENT

Prevention of diabetic nephropathy must focus on the metabolic and hemodynamic abnormalities that contribute to the progression of the kidney damage. Prevention of nephropathy can begin at the time of diagnosis of diabetes by optimizing glucose control. The Diabetes Control and Complications Trial demonstrated that intensive treatment to achieve tight glucose control reduced the risk of microalbuminuria by 34 percent ($p < 0.001$) and the risk of albuminuria by 56 percent ($p = 0.01$) in patients with Type I diabetes mellitus.[10] Although many practitioners believe that similar risk reductions will be achieved in Type II diabetes, this has yet to be proven. In order to achieve this level of meta-

bolic control, the ADA recommends glucose control with preprandial blood glucose concentrations of 80–120 mg/dl and target hemoglobin A_{1c} of 7 percent.[11] Similarly, reduction in dietary protein intake (0.6 gm/kg/day) may reduce urinary protein excretion and possibly slow the rate of decline in renal function.[12] Restricting dietary protein intake to less than 0.8 gm/kg/day (10% of total calories) is recommended for patients with overt proteinuria.

Pharmacologic measures to prevent diabetic nephropathy should focus on controlling systemic blood pressure and intraglomerular pressure. By lowering mean arterial pressure with antihypertensives, the pressure transmitted through the afferent arteriole to the glomerulus will be reduced. Hence, Joint National Committee (JNC) V recommends lowering blood pressure to less than 130/85 mmHg in patients with diabetes mellitus.[13] However, patients with early diabetic nephropathy and proteinuria may have elevated glomerular pressures prior to the development of systemic hypertension.[3,7] Angiotensin converting enzyme (ACE) inhibitors selectively reduce intraglomerular pressure by decreasing the formation of angiotensin-II and, thereby, dilating the efferent arteriole. The clinical benefits of ACE inhibitors have been evaluated in patients in various stages of diabetic nephropathy.

Evaluating ACE Inhibitors

In order to evaluate the effect of ACE inhibitors on progression of diabetic nephropathy, Lewis et al. performed a randomized, double-blind, placebo-controlled study of captopril 25 mg three times daily in patients with Type I diabetes mellitus with or without hypertension and Stage IV nephropathy (urinary protein > 500 mg/day) and serum creatinine < 2.5 mg/dL.[14] Over the median follow-up period of three years, the proportion of patients with a doubling of serum creatinine was 25/207 in the captopril group and 43/202 in the control group ($p = 0.007$). This represents a 48 percent reduction in risk with the use of captopril (95% CI:16%–69%). Similarly, the risk of death, dialysis, or renal transplantation was significantly reduced 50 percent (95% CI:18%–70%) in patients receiving captopril. Subgroup analysis revealed statistically significant reductions only for those patients with serum creatinine greater than 1.5 mg/dL. This study suggests that captopril slows the progressive decline in renal function in patients with Type I diabetes mellitus and established nephropathy.

Initiation of therapy earlier in the course of diabetic nephropathy may be more likely to substantially alter the rate of disease progression. The European Microalbuminuria Captopril Study evaluated the effect of captopril on progression to overt proteinuria in normotensive patients with Type I diabetes mellitus and microalbuminuria.[15] Patients were randomized to captopril 50 mg twice daily or placebo and followed for 24 months. Mean albumin excretion increased from 52 to 76 mcg/min (+18.3%) in the control group while decreasing from 52 to 41 mcg/min (–2.1%) in patients receiving captopril (p < 0.01). Significantly fewer patients progressed to overt proteinuria in the captopril group compared to controls (5% vs. 23%, p < 0.05). These data suggest that the use of ACE inhibitors in patients with Type I diabetes and microalbuminuria (Stage III) decreases proteinuria and prevents the progression of diabetic nephropathy.

While patients with Type I diabetes mellitus are more likely to develop nephropathy, the higher prevalence of Type II diabetes leads to a greater number of patients developing nephropathy from Type II diabetes. In order to evaluate the effect of ACE inhibitors on the progression of diabetic nephropathy, Ravid et al. performed a long-term study of enalapril in normotensive patients with Type II diabetes and microalbuminuria.[16] Patients were randomized to receive placebo or enalapril 10 mg once daily. At a five-year follow-up, 6/49 (12%) of patients receiving enalapril developed overt proteinuria compared to 19/45 (42%) (absolute risk reduction 30%, 95% CI 15%–45%). The rate of decline in renal function was significantly greater in the placebo group than in the enalapril group following two years of therapy.

In a subsequent two-year follow-up study, 94 patients were randomized to either continue therapy with enalapril or placebo or switch from enalapril to placebo or from placebo to enalapril.[17] The risk of developing overt proteinuria over seven years was significantly lower for patients receiving enalapril (18%) compared to placebo (60%) for the entire seven-year period (p < 0.001). The beneficial effect on renal function also persisted in the enalapril group. The addition of enalapril to patients previously treated with placebo stabilized proteinuria and serum creatinine. Sano et al. found similar benefits on proteinuria in both normotensive and hypertensive patients with Type II diabetes treated with enalapril for four years.[18] Renal function remained stable in all study groups. These studies suggest that enalapril has a long-term stabilizing effect on proteinuria and progression of diabetic nephropathy in normotensive and hypertensive patients with Type II diabetes.

Evaluating Calcium Channel Blockers

In some cases, patients are unable to tolerate ACE inhibitors or require alternative antihypertensive agents. In a randomized, crossover trial, Bakris compared the effects of diltiazem and lisinopril on nephrotic-range proteinuria in patients with Type II diabetes and hypertension.[19] Patients received six weeks of diltiazem or lisinopril with two-week baseline and washout periods. Proteinuria decreased from 4.1 g/day at baseline to 2.6 g/day during the initial lisinopril treatment period and 2.8 g/day during the initial diltiazem treatment period. Similar results occurred during the crossover period. There were no significant differences in arterial pressure, serum creatinine, or urinary protein between diltiazem and lisinopril. This suggests short-term use of diltiazem may provide benefits on proteinuria similar to lisinopril in patients with Type II diabetes and hypertension.

In a blinded, placebo-controlled trial, Mimran and colleagues compared the short-term effects of nifedipine SR 20 mg twice daily and captopril 25 mg twice daily in normotensive patients with Type

I diabetes and microalbuminuria.[20] After six weeks, mean urinary albumin excretion remained stable in the placebo group (97 and 95 mcg/min), decreased from 86 to 51 mcg/min in the captopril group, and increased from 86 to 122 mcg/min in the nifedipine group. This suggests that short-term use of nifedipine may worsen proteinuria. The long-term effects on progression of diabetic nephropathy were not evaluated.

In order to evaluate different types of calcium channel blockers in diabetic nephropathy, Demarie and Bakris compared the effects of diltiazem and nifedipine on proteinuria in 14 patients with Type II diabetes, hypertension, proteinuria, and mild renal insufficiency.[21] While mean proteinuria significantly decreased from 2.7 to 1.3 g/day in patients receiving diltiazem (p = 0.022), it significantly increased from 2.8 to 5.3 g/day in the nifedipine group (p = 0.022). Serum creatinine significantly increased in patients receiving nifedipine, but remained unchanged in patients receiving diltiazem. Nifedipine increases glomerular capillary pressure due to potent afferent arteriolar vasodilation, in contrast to diltiazem that reduces glomerular capillary pressure by vasodilatation of the efferent arteriole.[22] Although nicardipine is a dihydropyridine calcium antagonist like nifedipine, it does not appear to have detrimental effects on diabetic nephropathy.[23]

Slataper evaluated the effects of lisinopril, diltiazem, and atenolol with furosemide in patients with Type II diabetes mellitus, hypertension, and proteinuria.[24] After 18 months of therapy, albumin excretion decreased from 3.3 to 1.9 g/day (p < 0.05) with lisinopril, from 2.9 to 1.6 g/day (p < 0.05) with diltiazem, and from 3.1 to 2.9 g/day (no significant difference) with atenolol/furosemide. The glomerular filtration rate was not significantly different after 18 months of treatment with lisinopril or diltiazem, but was significantly reduced in the atenolol/furosemide group. There were no significant differences between lisinopril and diltiazem. The rate of decline in renal function was inversely related to the reduction in proteinuria. This supports the use of albumin excretion as a monitoring tool for the efficacy of antihypertensive agents in patients with diabetic nephropathy.

Because many of these studies in diabetic nephropathy have enrolled small numbers of patients, Kasiske and colleagues evaluated the effects of various antihypertensive agents in patients with Type I and Type II diabetes using a meta-regression analysis.[25] The effects of ACE inhibitors, calcium channel blockers, beta blockers, and "other agents" on blood pressure, glomerular filtration rate, proteinuria, and albuminuria were evaluated. Although ACE inhibitors and calcium channel blockers had a more positive effect on glomerular filtration rate, there were no significant differences among the various regimens. However, ACE inhibitors were the only class of agents that positively affected renal function independently of the effect on blood pressure. ACE inhibitors reduced proteinuria to a greater extent than other antihypertensives. This meta-analysis supports the use of ACE inhibitors as the antihypertensive of choice in patients with diabetic nephropathy.

COMBINATION THERAPY

Because ACE inhibitors and calcium channel blockers have each been found to have beneficial effects in patients with diabetic nephropathy, the role of combination therapy should be considered. Bakris and colleagues compared the effects of an ACE inhibitor and a calcium channel blocker each alone or in combination in 30 patients with hypertension, Type II diabetes mellitus, and nephrotic-range proteinuria (> 3.5 g/day).[26] Patients were randomized and titrated to receive lisinopril (mean dose 29 mg/day), verapamil sustained-release (mean dose 362 mg/day), lisinopril (mean dose 16 mg/day) plus verapamil (mean dose 187 mg/day), or hydrochlorothiazide (mean dose 19 mg/day) plus guanfacine (mean dose 2 mg/day) for 12 months. Mean urinary protein excretion significantly decreased from 5.9 to 2.5 g/day (p < 0.05) in the lisinopril group, from 5.7 to 2.9 g/day (p < 0.05) in the verapamil group, and from 6.8 to 1.7 g/day (p < 0.05) in the lisinopril/verapamil combination group, but minimally changed from 5.1 to 4.5 g/day (no significant difference) in the hydrochlorothiazide/guanfacine group. Combination therapy with lisinopril/verapamil had a significantly greater reduction in proteinuria than the other three groups. The rate of decline in GFR over the 12-month period was significantly greater for the patients receiving lisinopril alone compared to verapamil or the lower dose combination. This study suggests that some patients with established nephropathy may benefit from lower doses of combination therapy rather than higher doses of an ACE inhibitor.

In order to evaluate the role of combination therapy in patients with microalbuminuria, Fioretto et al. performed a sequential crossover evaluation of three months of therapy with the ACE inhibitor cilazapril, verapamil, and the combination in 16 patients with hypertension, Type II diabetes mellitus, and microalbuminuria.[27] Urinary albumin decreased from 180 mcg/min at baseline to 93 mcg/min ($p < 0.01$) with cilazapril, to 139 mcg/min ($p < 0.05$) with verapamil, and 41 mcg/min ($p < 0.01$) with combination therapy. Combination therapy produced a statistically greater reduction in proteinuria than either agent alone ($p < 0.05$). This study suggests that patients with earlier stages of diabetic nephropathy may benefit from combination therapy of an ACE inhibitor and a calcium channel blocker. Larger, long-term studies are still needed to further evaluate the place of combination therapy.

• • •

Patients with diabetes mellitus are commonly encountered in many clinical practice settings. In order to significantly reduce a patient's risk for the development of diabetic nephropathy, a systematic approach to the assessment of proteinuria and kidney function and management of abnormalities is necessary (Figure 3). Prevention and treatment of diabetic nephropathy begins with optimizing glucose control. Because microalbuminuria is a strong predictor of progressive diabetic nephropathy, patients should be monitored annually. It is also important to identify hypertension; therefore, annual screening of blood pressure is also recommended. For patients who develop hypertension, microalbuminuria, or proteinuria, ACE inhibitors are recommended as first-line antihypertensive agents. Other agents, particularly non-dihydropyridine calcium channel blockers, may be added to adequately control blood pressure to less than 130/85 mmHg. Close attention to all of these factors may reduce the incidence of this most common cause of end-stage renal disease.

REFERENCES

1. U.S. Renal Data System: *USRDS 1993 Annual Data Report.* National Institutes of Health, Bethesda, MD, March 1993.

2. Selby, J.V., et al. "The Natural History and Epidemiology of Diabetic Nephropathy: Implications for Prevention and Control." *Journal of the American Medical Association* 263, no. 14 (1990): 1,954–60.

3. Cziraky, M.J., et al. "Current Issues in Treating the Hypertensive Patient with Diabetes: Focus on Diabetic Nephropathy." *The Annals of Pharmacotherapy* 30 (1996): 791–801.

4. Nelson, R.G., et al. "Development and Progression of Renal Disease in Pima Indians with Non–Insulin Dependent Diabetes Mellitus." *New England Journal of Medicine* 335, no. 22 (1996): 1,636–42.

5. Krolewski, A.S. "The Natural History of Diabetic Nephropathy in Type I Diabetes and the Role of Hypertension," pp 795–98. In Noth, R.H. "Diabetic Nephropathy: Hemodynamic Basis and Implications for Disease Management." *Annals of Internal Medicine* 110, no. 10 (1989): 795–813.

6. Brancati, F.L., et al. "The Excess Incidence of Diabetic End-Stage Renal Disease According to Race and Type of Diabetes." *Journal of the American Medical Association* 268, (1992): 3,079–84.

7. Kaysen, G.A. "Proteinuria as a Marker of Glomerular Injury," pp 798–802. In Noth, RH. "Diabetic Nephropathy: Hemodynamic Basis and Implications for Disease Management." *Annals of Internal Medicine* 110, no. 10 (1989): 795–813.

8. Laffel, L.M.B., et al. "The Impact of Blood Pressure on Renal Function in Insulin-Dependent Diabetes." (abstract) *Kidney International* 31 (1987): 207.

9. American Diabetes Association Consensus Statement. "Diagnosis and Management of Nephropathy in Patients with Diabetes Mellitus." *Diabetes Care* 19, Supplement 1 (1996): S103–S106.

10. The Diabetes Control and Complications Trial Research Group. "The Effect of Intensive Treatment of Diabetes on the Development and Progression of Long-term Complications in Insulin-Dependent Diabetes Mellitus." *New England Journal of Medicine* 329, no. 14 (1993): 977–86.

11. American Diabetes Association Position Statement. "Standards of Medical Care for Patients with Diabetes Mellitus." *Diabetes Care* 19, Supplement 1, (1996): S8–S15.

12. Brouhard, B.H., and LaGrone, L. "Effect of Dietary Protein Restriction on Functional Renal Reserve in Diabetic Nephropathy." *American Journal of Medicine* 89 (October 1990): 427–31.

13. Joint National Committee. "The Fifth Report of the Joint National Committee on Detection, Evaluation, and Treatment of High Blood Pressure." *Archives of Internal Medicine* 153 (1993): 154–83.

14. Lewis, E.J., et al. "The Effect of Angiotensin-Converting Enzyme Inhibition on Diabetic Nephropathy." *New England Journal of Medicine* 329, no. 20 (1993): 1,456–62.

15. Vibeti, G., et al. "Effect of Captopril Progression to Clinical Proteinuria in Patients with Insulin-Dependent Diabetes Mellitus and Microalbuminuria." *Journal of the American Medical Association* 271, no. 4 (1994): 275–79.

16. Ravid, M., et al. "Long-Term Stabilizing Effect of Angiotensin-Converting Enzyme Inhibition on Plasma Creatinine and on Proteinuria in Normotensive Type II Diabetic Patients." *Annals of Internal Medicine* 118, no. 8, (1993): 577–81.

17. Ravid, M., et al. "Long-term Renoprotective Effect of Angiotensin-Converting Enzyme Inhibition in Non-insulin-dependent Diabetes Mellitus: A 7-Year Follow-Up Study." *Archives of Internal Medicine* 156 (1996): 286–89.

18. Sano, T., et al. "Effects of Long-Term Enalapril Treatment on Persistent Microalbuminuria in Well-Controlled Hypertensive and Normotensive NIDDM Patients." *Diabetes Care* 17, no. 5 (1994): 420–24.

19. Bakris, G.L. "Effects of Diltiazem or Lisinopril on Massive Proteinuria Associated with Diabetes Mellitus." *Annals of Internal Medicine* 112, no. 9 (1990): 707–08.

20. Mimran, A., et al. "Comparative Effect of Captopril and Nifedipine in Normotensive Patients with Incipient Diabetic Nephropathy." *Diabetes Care* 11, no. 10 (1988): 850–53.

21. Demarie, B.K, and Bakris, G.L. "Effects of Different Calcium Antagonists on Proteinuria Associated with Diabetes Mellitus." *Annals of Internal Medicine* 113, no. 12 (1990): 987–88.

22. Valentino, V.A., et al. "A Perspective on Converting Enzyme Inhibitors and Calcium Channel Antagonists in Diabetic Renal Disease." *Archives of Internal Medicine* 151 (1991): 2,367–72.

23. Baba, T., et al. "Renal Effects of Nicardipine, a Calcium Entry Blocker, in Hypertensive Type II Diabetic Patients with Nephropathy." *Diabetes* 35 (1986): 1,206–14.

24. Slataper, R., et al. "Comparative Effects of Different Antihypertensive Treatments on Progression of Diabetic Renal Disease." *Archives of Internal Medicine* 153 (1993): 973–80.

25. Kasiske, B.L., et al. "Effect of Antihypertensive Therapy on the Kidney in Patients with Diabetes: A Meta-Regression Analysis." *Annals of Internal Medicine* 118, no. 2 (1993): 129–38.

26. Bakris, G.L., Barnhill, B.W., and Sadler, R. "Treatment of Arterial Hypertension in Diabetic Humans: Importance of Therapeutic Selection." *Kidney International* 41 (1992): 912–19.

27. Fioretto, P., et al. "Effects of Angiotensin Converting Enzyme Inhibitors and Calcium Antagonists on Atrial Natriuretic Peptide Release and Action and on Albumin Excretion Rate in Hypertensive Insulin-Dependent Diabetic Patients." *American Journal of Hypertension* 5 (1992): 837–46.

CHAPTER 4

Managing the Care of the Diabetic Transplant Patient

Jerry Siegel, RPh, FASHP, Victoria S. DeVore, PharmD, and
Sue M. Bosley, PharmD

Care of the diabetic transplant patient presents many challenges for therapeutic manage-ment. Complications of diabetes such as retinopathy, neuropathy, hyperglycemia, and hypertension add to the already difficult management of nondiabetic transplant patients. The role of the pharmacist as an educator, counselor, and interaction and profile manager is an essential part of a successful transplant program. Understanding the purpose of the medications and their side effects is vital for the patient to comply with a demanding medication regimen. This depth of understanding cannot be conveyed without repetitive educational efforts that are reinforced by all of the health care practitioners and supportive family members. Although kidney transplantation offers freedom from dialysis, it does not offer freedom from insulin dependence. Kidney–pancreas, pancreas, or islet cell transplan-tation may provide insulin independence and are the only curative interventions available. Evaluation of the research literature compares the advantages and complications of these surgical modalities. Early intervention with transplantation may offer insulin-dependent diabetics a new opportunity to improve their quality of life; however, intensive educational efforts and assurance of compliance are essential for successful outcomes. Key words: *diabetes mellitus, diabetic neuropathy, islet cell, kidney–pancreas transplant, kidney transplant, patient education, retinopathy, transplant pharmacist*

INTRODUCTION

After three years of educating transplant pa-tients about their medications, I faced my great-est challenge. A 29-year-old male post–kidney transplant patient was ready for education. The problem he presented was that he was a juvenile onset (Type I) diabetic patient who was blind, illiterate, and had severe peripheral neuropathy. The patient lived with his mother in a trailer and since she worked, he needed to have a signifi-cant amount of independence.

Normally blind patients can be taught to iden-tify their medicine bottles by cutting felt shapes into letters that correspond with the names of the medicines. If the patient is illiterate, the shapes can be simply different numbers of felt stripes, and the patient must remember the correspond-ing numbers. This patient had peripheral neur-opathy from the diabetes and could not distin-guish the number of stripes and did not know the alphabet. He was able to open the non–child-proof containers and with difficulty could sepa-rate and count out his pills. What he needed was a way to identify his bottles. Since he could hear and smell, the education was focused around those senses.

A vial containing cotton impregnated with a smell was made and associated with characteris-tics of the medication that the patient could re-member. For example, wild cherry was associ-ated with the patient's digoxin tablets since the patient could relate the color red to both cherries and the heart. A hickory-smoked smell reminded the patient of smoked ham, a food item that was not allowed because of the salt content. This was attached to the patient's furosemide tablets. Peppermint smell was attached to the azathioprine since it was taken once a day in the "PM."

The patient was not able to draw up his own insulin, but I was able to teach him to inject his thigh with a predrawn syringe by using his wrist to press down on the plunger. His mother was able to draw up his insulin.

He had a general sense of telling time by either shows on television or the dials on an open clock. I made a board that had a clock face and a single movable hand. At the 12, 3, 6, and 9 o'clock positions, holes were drilled to hold the bottles corresponding with the medication bottles that were due that particular time. In this way, both the sense of smell and the clock position could be used for identification. This was important since he was not able to see or feel the individual tablets.

After nearly a month of training, the patient was able to master his medication program and go home. The year was 1979, there were no home care programs, and the family wished to remain independent. Although they were very poor they did not receive "welfare" and resisted any form of charity.

Even though the patient did well for several years, this case left more than just a distinctive memory. The patient worked very hard to gain some degree of independence, and sometimes we may forget the importance of this in education and have a tendency to do everything for the patient.

The diabetic patient has many challenges to face, as illustrated by this case, and the challenges for management can sometimes seem overwhelming. The diabetic patient today has more options for health care and more advanced technology medications and even types of insulin. However, the disease process remains the same and the educational challenges are not that much different than in 1979.

TRANSPLANTATION FOR TREATMENT OF DIABETES

The only option to "cure" Type I diabetes mellitus is transplantation. Kidney–pancreas, pancreas after kidney, pancreas alone, or islet cell transplantation are all methods that have been used to eliminate the need for insulin injections. With the advents of these newer surgical techniques, the option for transplantation may not have to be reserved for end-stage renal disease. The devastations of long-term diabetes are not reversed by transplantation, so early intervention may be essential to prevent irreversible damage.

Education for the transplant patient is also not a one-time intervention but a system of support over a lifetime. The role of the pharmacist has shifted to an ambulatory setting as the length of stay of the patient has decreased to less than seven days. The ambulatory pharmacist has become a consultant, an educator, and a manager for the complicated regimen of medications that are part of the transplant patient's life.

CURRENT SUCCESS IN SOLID ORGAN TRANSPLANTATION

Solid organ transplantation has been hailed as the treatment of choice for patients with end-stage renal failure.[1-4] The shortage of available organs is the major limitation on expanding this treatment option. Although pancreas transplants are being performed with increasing numbers in patients with Type I diabetes, the majority are in conjunction with a kidney transplant.[5,6] Transplantation of islet cells is not a new concept. The theory behind islet cells transplantation is the potential cure for insulin-dependent diabetes.[7,8] Data from the United Network for Organ Sharing (UNOS), as of November 1994, report that 34,212 patients are on the waiting list for a kidney transplant, 318 for a pancreas, 1,488 for a kidney–pancreas, and 55 for a pancreas islet cells transplant. In addition, from January 1 to December 1995, 10,892 kidneys (3,208 living related donors), 110 pancreas, and 918 kidney–

pancreas transplants were performed.[5] Based on information from the International Islet Transplant Registry, 215 islet cells transplants have been performed worldwide since 1993.[6]

The differences in the type of transplant correlate significantly with the graft survival probability. In addition, the surgical technique and potential postoperative complications have a tremendous impact on the overall allograft survival rate. Survival rates for kidney transplants vary depending if the donor is a living related or a cadaver. The overall one-year graft survival rate for kidney cadaveric was reported at 76 to 89 percent.[1,9–11] The one-year survival rate for living related kidney transplants exceeds 90 percent and is as high as 99 percent from a few studies.[1,3,5,12] Transplants with a greater survival rate have been attributed to better human leukocyte antigen matching, early posttransplant function, and increased experience with immunosuppressive regimens.[9,10,12–15]

The majority of pancreas transplantation is in conjunction with a kidney transplantation. However, pancreas transplantation may be an option for patients with insulin-dependent diabetes, who may or may not have preexisting renal dysfunction. The goal of pancreas transplantation is to prevent the progression or occurrence of secondary complications associated with diabetes.[16] However, support from the literature is not consistent.[17–22] Although there is a higher risk associated with kidney–pancreas transplantation, the overall graft survival is higher than with pancreas transplant alone.[23] The fairly dismal overall graft survival for pancreas transplant alone was 49 percent in one reported study, 45 percent when a kidney had previously been transplanted, and 75 percent with a simultaneous kidney–pancreas transplant.[24] An additional study reported a one-year pancreas graft survival rate of 72 to 79 percent, compared with kidney–pancreas at 91 percent.[25] In other recent studies, the investigators reported a success rate of 89 percent in pancreas-alone transplantation.[1,24] Contributing factors for the inconsistent success in graft survival rate may be due to postsurgical complications,

immunosuppressive regimens, and favorable patient selection.[23,26]

Due to the continual shortage of available organs, an alternative approach in improving glucose control may be islet cell transplantation. Current data on insulin independence at one year for islet cell transplantation were reported at 45 percent to 51 percent.[7,8] Possible limiting factors for preventing engraftment may be due to the number of islets transplanted, immune rejection of the islets, and toxicity associated with immunosuppressive medications. Routine transplantation of islet cells does not seem practical due to the limiting factors listed. Nonhuman sources will most likely be a feasible alternative source for islet cells.[7,15,25]

The three types of pancreas transplantation are simultaneous kidney–pancreas, pancreas after kidney, and pancreas transplant alone. Usually the whole organ is transplanted; however, the tail may be transplanted instead.[27–30] There is not a common consensus on what is the best procedure to drain the exocrine secretions from the transplanted pancreas. The native pancreas is left intact; therefore, additional endocrine secretions are produced. In the past, there were three surgical procedures used; however, new information is available concerning a new approach.[6,27–30]

With the first approach, the pancreas duct is injected with a synthetic polymer glue to occlude. This procedure eliminates exocrine function, but causes a severe inflammatory process that may lead to fibrosis and damage islets. The second is enteric drainage that allows the exocrine secretions to drain into the loop of jejunum, which may lead to bacterial infections. The third is bladder drainage where a segment of the donor duodenum is connected to the pancreas and the bladder. Complications associated with bladder drainage are dehydration, acidosis, recurrent urinary tract infections, reflux graft pancreatitis, and hematuria. The newest approach is a portal venous drainage.[27] Portal venous drainage was associated with a significant decrease in acidosis and dehydration compared to bladder drainage.

Islet cells are isolated from the pancreas by using enzymes that digest the surrounding tissue. The islet cells are transplanted by a simple procedure that requires only a local anesthetic and a single injection. Examples of ways that islets may be transplanted include injection through the portal vein, intramuscular, or in the peritoneal cavity.[7,8,25] A limiting factor in the numbers of islet cell transplantations is the difficulty in obtaining a sufficient amount of islets for transplantation. A theory under investigation to improve outcome is the use of semipermeable membranes that would allow glucose, oxygen, and insulin to pass freely and prevent the components of the immune system to penetrate.[25]

Table 1 presents sources from the literature that document solid organ transplantation studies and results.

THE ROLES OF THE TRANSPLANT PHARMACIST

The role of a clinical pharmacist in the current health care environment has changed significantly. New positions and opportunities are available in the area of patient care. The pharmacist is now considered to be a very valuable member of the patient's care team. This role is very interactive and challenging. Clinical pharmacists are required to be experts in their particular field of practice. These expectations are no different for transplant pharmacists.

The transplant patient population is quite unique and complicated because of the number and type of medications these patients take. Prior to transplantation these patients have had long-standing chronic illnesses such as diabetes, hypertension, lupus, or renal failure requiring some form of dialysis. Some patients have little understanding or insight as to why they need to take so many different "pills" each and every day for the rest of their lives. Whether the patient receives a kidney, pancreas, liver, or kidney plus a pancreas, the survival of a successful transplant organ requires a full-time commitment of compliance by the patient. Patients may assume that once they actually are transplanted all of their medical problems will be over. Furthermore, the recipient of a kidney transplant may have a functioning kidney, but may still suffer from disease such as diabetes that continues to burden the patient's overall health. The new transplant becomes a life-saving treatment for these patients. It is obvious that the next most important job is to keep and retain the transplant for a long period of time. This takes a lot of effort, because the patient must be compliant with many medications and with being subjected to a large number of medical procedures.

The transplant population's medication profiles are very specialized in themselves. The transplant pharmacist must have a good working understanding of each of these medications and the roles that they play in the patient's therapy. The cornerstone to this patient group's therapy is the immunosuppressant agents. Included in this category are cyclosporin, azathioprine, tacrolimus (FK506), mycophenolate, and prednisone. Each one of these agents can inflict a gamut of side effects on the unsuspecting transplant recipient. Some of the more common side effects can be cyclosporin-induced hypertension and hirsutism; diarrhea caused by mycophenolate; and gastric ulcers and osteoporosis brought on by prednisone.[31,32]

Besides the immunosuppressants, many other auxiliary medications are generally required. Some of these medications are needed to counteract the side effects produced by the patient's immunosuppression. Antihypertensive agents are found in almost every transplant patient's profile. Many of these patients were hypertensive before their transplant and still require treatment, or patients may have developed hypertension secondary to their immunosuppression medications. All classes of antihypertensive agents can be utilized; however, they are not all used equally.

Angiotensin converting enzyme (ACE) inhibitors should be prescribed with caution in patients

Table 1. Literature support

Title	Years	Ref. no.	n	Type of transplant	Study design	Results
Long-term outcome of kidney–pancreas transplant recipients with good graft function at one year	1987–92	26	50	Kidney–pancreas	Pts. were assessed for graft survival, graft function, and progression of diabetic complications at 1 year and min. of 3-year follow-up	Five-year kidney survival reported at 85% and pancreas at 85%. The exocrine drainage for all pancreatic grafts was by duo-denocystomy. The authors reported that if graft is functioning after 1 year had a >85% chance of surviving at least 5 additional years.
Comparison before and after transplantation of pancreas–kidney and pancreas–kidney with loss of pancreas—A prospective controlled quality of life study	1992–94	16	38	Kidney–pancreas	Standardized home-based interview is done during dialysis and repeated 5, 12, and 18 months after transplantation. Quality of life (QoL) was evaluated in patients who received a pancreas–kidney transplantation (PKT) and whom the pancreas failed soon after transplantation (PKT-P). Quality of life was defined by the patient's perception of physical and occupational function, mental state, social interaction, and somatic sensation.	Both groups rated with QoL higher compared with dialysis. The PKT group QoL scored higher compared to the PKT-P group.
Success and complications of pancreatic transplantation at one institution	1987–92	23	59	Kidney–pancreas (47) Pancreas (12)	Retrospective review of the results and complications after combined kidney–pancreas (KP) and pancreas transplantation. The results were divided into era I (1987–92) and era II (1993–95).	<table><tr><td></td><td>Era I</td><td>Era II</td></tr><tr><td>Rej. episodes</td><td>76%</td><td>50%</td></tr><tr><td>Pt. survival</td><td>84%</td><td>91%</td></tr><tr><td>Pancreas survival</td><td>57%</td><td>79%</td></tr><tr><td>Kidney survival</td><td>89%</td><td>94%</td></tr><tr><td>KP survival</td><td>70%</td><td>90%</td></tr></table>

continues

Table 1. Continued

Title	Years	Ref. no.	n	Type of transplant	Study design	Results
Renal allograft and patient outcome after transplantation: Pancreas–kidney(PK) versus kidney-alone transplants in Type I diabetic patients (KA-D) versus kidney-alone in nondiabetic patients (KA-ND).	1988–94	1	204	PK (61) KA-D (63) KA-ND (80)	Retrospective review of renal allograft outcome based on the three groups of kidney transplants.	Overall decrease in rejection episodes and graft loss were attributed to the initial use of antilymphocyte antibody and quadruple-therapy immunosuppression therapy. The increased episodes of rejection in Era I are linked to the decreased graft survival in Era I. PK / KA-D / KA-ND # failed grafts 17(28%) 37(59%) 37(46%) Rejection 8(13%) 11(18%) 20(25%) 1 yr survival 82% 76% 89% 5 yr survival 69% 49% 63% PK transplantation associated with increased incidence of acute rejection of the renal allograft. Sepsis was more frequent cause of renal graft failure in the PK group. The higher pt. survival rate in the PK group probably reflects recipient selection bias.
Mortality of cadaveric kidney transplantation versus combined kidney–pancreas transplantation in diabetic patients	1987–93	11	100	Kidney–pancreas (54) Kidney (46)	Determine whether combined kidney–pancreas (KP) transplantation is associated with higher mortality than kidney transplantation alone (living rated-LRD and cadaveric-KTA)	KP / LRD / KTA 3-yr pt. survival 68% 86% 90% KP recipients had a higher rate of infectious deaths within the first 12 months.

who received kidney transplants, since hyperkalemia can occur when cyclosporin is given concurrently with these agents.[33,34] If an ACE inhibitor is needed, a low dose should be utilized. The patient must be made aware of the damaging effects of hypertension on the kidney, and the possibility of losing a transplant due to this. Because of the increased risk of infection induced by immunosuppression, the transplant patient is usually placed on a daily maintenance dose of an antibiotic. Common medications used for this purpose are sulfamethoxazole/trimethoprim, ciprofloxacin, amoxicillin, or sulfamethoxazole by itself.[35] Gastric ulcer prophylaxis is also needed to counteract the use of prednisone in these patients. Many patients are initially started on an antacid regimen consisting of aluminum/magnesium hydroxide preparations. If this is not sufficient, a histamine receptor antagonist (H_2) blocker or even an agent like omeprazole may be needed.[36]

Because of the vast changes pharmacy practice has gone through, it is evident that the clinical pharmacist will assume many new roles and not just one or two. Of course, these roles will continue to change and multiply as medical science advances. Some of the roles that a transplant pharmacist assumes are educator, interviewer, detective, counselor, confidant, and monitor. Each of these functions has its own importance that influences the patient's care. The clinical pharmacist has to remain flexible and willing to take on new challenges in order to meet the demands of an ever-changing environment. The following text will discuss pertinent roles donned by the transplant pharmacist.

Educator

The pharmacist acts in this capacity not only with the patients and their families, but also with other clinical staff, including physicians and nurses. It is imperative that patients understand all of their medications. Each patient on average takes 10 or more different medications a day. Just trying to remember to take their medications

is difficult; however, if patients do not know why they need them, they may believe it is alright to miss a few doses. The pharmacist must counsel each patient and his or her family members if possible. Patients must understand the purpose of each medication and why it is important that they continue the therapy. The staff expects a clinical pharmacist to be accessible and function as a resource of drug information for physicians and nurses.

Counselor/Confidant

Establishing patients' compliance is extremely critical, since they may actually be taking their medications quite differently than prescribed. An accurate medication history is essential. It is important to ask patients open-ended questions that do not lead them into saying what they perceive the pharmacist wants to hear. Ample time must be allowed to interview patients. The pharmacist must not assume patients understand everything that is told to them. Patients often feel more comfortable talking to a pharmacist. They feel the pharmacist has more time to answer their questions and focus on their concerns. During this contact, the pharmacist is able to access patients' general mood and attitude toward their care. It is a known fact that patients with chronic illnesses can suffer from depression. Depression can greatly hinder the patient's outcome to treatment. If the pharmacist notices any signs of depression such as decreased/increased appetite, lack of enthusiasm, or no desire to take his or her medications, it is imperative to start antidepressant therapy quickly. Depressed patients suffer a very poor quality of life.[37]

Drug Interaction Monitor

Because of the complex nature of this population's medication management, drug interactions and drug scheduling need to be continually monitored by the transplant pharmacist. As the number of medications taken by a patient increases, so does the likelihood of drug interactions. For example, cyclosporin blood levels are increased by ketoconazole, fluconazole, itraconazole, erythromycin, diltiazem, cimetidine, and oral contraceptives; however, rifampin, phenytoin, phenobarbital, carbamazepine, nafcillin, and octreotide decrease its activity.[38] Often the timing of the medications themselves is overlooked. Ketoconazole should be given after a meal to increase its absorption,[39] and the hydroxymethylglutary-CoA (HMG CoA) reductase inhibitors work more efficiently if given in the evening.[40] Antacid preparations can be very troublesome by decreasing the absorption of certain medications such as ciprofloracin or warfarin. These medications should be taken at least one to two hours apart, which can be difficult if the patient is taking an antacid every two hours.[41]

Patient Profile Manager

A wealth of information can be found in each patient's clinic chart. Reviewing these charts gives the pharmacist a broad picture of the patient's progress through the transplantation process. Important trends in the patient's overall condition can be identified through this type of a review. Drug level monitoring cannot be overlooked, since the physician sees this as one of the primary duties of a pharmacist. Some critical drugs to monitor through blood levels include cyclosporin, digoxin, and certain antibiotics such as aminoglycosides or vancomycin. The physician also relies on the pharmacist to perform any pharmacokinetic calculations that need to be done.

Patient Care Manager

The pharmacist may be called upon to perform other duties that are not as traditional as drug monitoring, but still influence the pharmaceutical care of the patient. For instance, problems can arise when patients do not receive the correct medication or strength from their personal pharmacy. This problem has occurred with some mail-order pharmacies. Higher strengths, which are often difficult to break, may be sent for cost savings.

The pharmacist may also be called upon to make clarifications with other clinicians who care for the transplant patient. This involvement can include writing to physicians in order to make sure they know the patient's current medication profile, or even calling in new prescriptions to the patient's pharmacy in order to ensure that the patient will be obtaining the correct medication and strength.

Specialist Therapy Designer

The pharmacist has to target special patient populations to ensure they understand their medication therapy. Some of these populations include patients who are blind, hearing impaired, mentally challenged, illiterate, or have lost peripheral senses due to diabetic neuropathy. These populations need more specialized counseling to ensure they will take their medications properly. The patients' support system can play a large role in their care. Spouses, parents, siblings, or friends can be very helpful sources of information, and they also may be highly involved in the patients' care.

•   •   •

The unfortunate patient from the 1979 transplant program would clearly have benefited from the advances in surgical and medical modalities of the 1990s. Early kidney–pancreas transplantation may have afforded not only insulin independence but also possibly reduction of the risk of retinopathy that led to total blindness. Early islet cell transplantation may have prevented the diabetic nephropathy that led to end-stage renal disease. Despite the advances in transplantation and immunosuppressive therapy, however, lack of compliance with these complicated regimens still would lead to organ failure and advance of the diabetic disease process. A multidisciplinary approach to patient care is essential to a successful outcome and the role of the pharmacist in both the acute care and ambulatory setting is necessary to achieve optimal results. The next decade may promote disease state management protocols that provide cost-effective interventions with islet cell transplantation, insulin independence, and substantially improved quality of life.

REFERENCES

1. Douzdjian, V., et al. "Renal Allograft and Patient Outcomes after Transplantation: Pancreas–Kidney versus Kidney-Alone Transplants in Type 1 Diabetic Patients versus Kidney-Alone Transplants in Nondiabetic Patients." *American Journal of Kidney Diseases* 27, no. 1 (1996): 106–16.

2. Haberal, M., et al. "Kidney Transplantation at One Center: 1-Year Results." *Transplantation Proceedings* 28, no. 1 (1996): 410–11.

3. Schaubel, D., et al. "Survival Experience among Elderly End-Stage Renal Disease Patients." *Transplantation* 60, no. 12 (1995): 1,389–94.

4. Karlber, I., and Nyber, G. "Cost-Effectiveness Studies of Renal Transplantation." *International Journal of Technology Assessment in Health Care* 11, no. 3 (1995): 611–22.

5. "United Network for Organ Sharing (UNOS) Registry." 1987. [electronic bulletin board].204.127.237.11/usd11_20.htm. Available from listserv@http://www.unos.com

6. Stratta, R.J., et al. "Pancreas Transplantation." *Renal Failure* 17, no. 4 (1995): 323–37.

7. Wahoff, D.C., et al. "Autologous Islet Transplantation to Prevent Diabetes after Pancreatic Resection." *Annals of Surgery* 222, no. 4 (1995): 562–79.

8. Brunicardi, F.C., et al. "Clinical Islet Transplantation Experience of the University of California Islet Transplant Consortium." *Surgery* 118, (1995): 967–72.

9. Najarian, J.S., et al. "The Impact of the Quality of Initial Graft Function on Cadaver Kidney Transplants." *Transplantation* 57, no. 6 (1994): 812–16.

10. Troppmann, C., et al. "Delayed Graft Function, Acute Rejection, and Outcome after Cadaver Renal Transplantation." *Transplantation* 59, no. 7 (1995): 962–68.

11. Cheung, A., et al. "Simultaneous Pancreas–Kidney Transplant versus Kidney Transplant Alone in Diabetic Patients." *Kidney International* 41, (1992): 924–29.

12. Manske, C.L., Wang, Y., and Thomas, W. "Mortality of Cadaveric Kidney Transplantation versus Combined Kidney–Pancreas Transplantation in Diabetic Patients." *Lancet* 346, (1995): 1,658–62.

13. Mital, D., et al. "Renal Transplantation without Sutures Using the Vascular Clipping System for Renal Artery and Vein Anastomosis—A New Technique." *Transplantation* 62, no. 8 (1996): 1,171–73.

14. Patrasi, G.M., et al. "Reduced Fibrinolytic Potential One Year after Kidney Transplantation." *Transplantation* 59, no. 10 (1995): 1,416–20.

15. Danovitch, G.M. *Handbook of Kidney Transplantation.* 2d ed. Boston: Little Brown, 1996.

16. Adang, E.M., et al. "Comparison before and after Transplantation of Pancreas–Kidney and Pancreas–Kidney with Loss of Pancreas—A Prospective Controlled Quality of Life Study." *Transplantation* 62, no. 6 (1996): 754–58.

17. Kennedy, W.R., et al. "Effects of Pancreatic Transplantation on Diabetic Neuropathy." *New England Journal of Medicine* 322, no. 15 (1990): 322–37.

18. Ramsey, R.C., et al. "Progression of Diabetic Retinopathy after Pancreas Transplantation for Insulin-Dependent Diabetes Mellitus." *New England Journal of Medicine* 318, no. 4 (1988): 208–14.

19. Zehr, P.S., et al. "Pancreas Transplantation: Assessing Secondary Complications and Life Quality." *Diabetolgia* 34 (1991): S138–40.

20. Zehr, C.L. and Gross, C.R. "Quality of Life of Pancreas Transplant Recipients." *Diabetolgia* 34 (1991): S145–49.

21. Solders, G., et al. "Effects of Combined Pancreatic and Renal Transplantation on Diabetic Neuropathy: A Two-Year Follow-Up Study." *Lancet* (1987): 1,232–35.

22. Bohman, S.O., et al. "Recurrent Diabetic Nephropathy in Renal Allografts Placed in Diabetic Patients and Protective Effect of Simultaneous Pancreatic Transplantation." *Transplantation Proceedings* 19, no. 1 (1987): 2,290–93.

23. Jones, J.W., Mizrahi, S.S., and Bently, F.R. "Success and Complications of Pancreatic Transplantation at One Institution." *Annals of Surgery* 223, no. 6 (1996): 757–64.

24. Kinkhabwala, M., et al. "The Role of Whole Organ Pancreas Transplantation in the Treatment of Type I Diabetes." *American Journal of Surgery* 171 (1996): 516–20.

25. Sun, Y., et al. "Normalization of Diabetes in Spontaneously Diabetic Cynomologus Monkeys by Xenografts of Microencapsulated Porcine Islets without Immunosuppression." *Journal of Clinical Investigation* 98, no. 6 (1996): 1,417–22.

26. Bruce, D.S., et al. "Long-Term Outcome of Kidney–Pancreas Transplant Recipients with Good Graft Function at One Year." *Transplantation* 62, no. 4 (1996): 451–56.

27. Newell, K.A., et al. "Comparison of Pancreas Transplantation with Portal Venous and Enteric Exocrine Drainage to the Standard Technique Utilizing Bladder Drainage of Exocrine Secretions." *Transplantation* 62, no. 9 (1996): 1,353–56.

28. Sollinger, H.W., et al. "Experience with 100 Consecutive Simultaneous Kidney–Pancreas Transplants with Bladder Drainage." *Annals of Surgery* 214, no. 6 (1991): 703–11.

29. Schwartz, S.I. "Transplantation." In *Principles of Surgery,* edited by S.I. Schwartz, et al. New York: McGraw-Hill, 1994.

30. Dupuis, R.E. "Solid Organ Transplantation." In *Applied Therapeutics: The Clinical Use of Drugs.* 6th ed. edited by L.Y. Young. Vancouver, WA: Applied Therapeutics, 1995.

31. Johnson, R.W. "Primary Regimens in Immunosuppression." *Nephrology, Dialysis, Transplantation* 10 [Suppl. 1] (1995): 101–04.

32. Yun, Y.S., et al. "Changes of Bone Metabolism Indices in Patients Receiving Immunosuppressive Therapy Including Low Doses of Steroids after Renal Transplantation." *Transplantation Proceedings* 28, no. 3 (1996): 1,561–64.

33. Pei, Y., et al. "Extrarenal Effect of Cyclosporin A on Potassium Homeostasis in Renal Transplant Recipients." *American Journal of Kidney Diseases* 22, no. 2 (1993): 314–19.

34. Schlueter, W., Keilani, T., and Batlle, D.C. "Tissue Renin Angiotensin Systems: Theoretical Implications for the Development of Hyperkalemia Using Angiotensin-Converting Enzyme Inhibitors." *American Journal of the Medical Sciences* 307 [Suppl. 1] (1994): S81–86.

35. Ko, K.S., et al. "Infections after Renal Transplantation." *Transplantation Proceedings* 26, no. 4 (1994): 2,072–74.

36. Grino, J.M., et al. "Antilymphoblast Globulin, Cyclosporin, and Steroids in Cadaveric Renal Transplantation." *Transplantation* 49 (1990): 1,114–17.

37. Kiley, D.J., Lam, C.S., and Pollak, R. "A Study of Treatment Compliance Following Kidney Transplantation." *Transplantation* 55, no. 1 (1993): 51–56.

38. Yee, G.C. "Pharmacokinetic Interactions between Cyclosporin and Other Drugs." *Transplantation Proceedings* 22, no. 3 (1990): 1,203–07.

39. Symoens, J., et al. "An Evaluation of Two Years of Clinical Experience with Ketoconazole." *Reviews of Infectious Diseases* 2, no. 4 (1980): 674–87.

40. Illingworth, D.R. "Comparative Efficacy of Once Versus Twice Daily Mevinolin in the Therapy of Familial Hypercholesterolemia." *Clinical Pharmacology and Therapeutics* 40, no. 3 (1986): 338–43.

41. Teixeira, M.H., et al. "Complexes of Ciprofloxacin with Metal Ions Contained in Antacid Drugs." *Journal of Chemotherapy* 7, no. 2 (1995): 126–32.

CHAPTER 5

Applying the Principles of Pharmaceutical Care to the Patient with Diabetes

Richard Segal, PhD

Current medical care for patients with diabetes neither meets the guidelines from the American Diabetes Association (ADA) nor approaches the levels of intensive care in the Diabetes Control and Complications Trial (DCCT). The drug-use process for patients with diabetes could be enhanced by improving the way in which drug therapy is monitored and managed. The concept of pharmaceutical care strategically redefines the drug-use process into a pharmaceutical care system in which the pharmacist takes responsibility for monitoring the effects of drugs and acts to resolve drug-related problems before they become a drug-related morbidity. A method for implementing a pharmaceutical care service using practice guidelines to help a pharmacist provide consistent care to all patients with diabetes is discussed. Key words: *diabetes, monitoring, pharmaceutical care*

While the present drug-use process has many obvious strengths, it could be improved. The weaknesses of the current drug-use process, the role of pharmaceutical care in improving the drug-use process, and specific suggestions for implementing a pharmaceutical care service for the patient with diabetes are covered in this article.

THE CURRENT DRUG USE PROCESS

The current drug-use process typically begins with a patient recognizing that he or she has a medical problem requiring a visit with the primary care physician. During the physician–patient encounter, subjective and objective data are routinely collected about the patient's condition, followed by an analysis of the data. The encounter usually concludes with the development and implementation of a therapeutic plan. The therapeutic plan can include setting explicit objectives for the patient and prescribing a medication. In the community setting, the pharmacist's role in the present drug-use process usually starts when the patient brings a drug prescription to the pharmacy, at which point the pharmacist reviews the prescription, dispenses the medication, and may provide advice to the patient.

While the current drug-use process works well for many patients, a significant number of patients do not reach their therapeutic objectives. Some patients even experience a drug-related morbidity. Typically, 4 to 5 percent of all hospitalizations are a result of drug-related morbidity, and perhaps as many as 50 percent of those morbidities could have been prevented if the drug-use process had been working better.[1] Considerable evidence is showing the unnecessary social and economic costs resulting from drug-related morbidity. Economic analyses suggest that for every dollar spent on purchasing pharmaceuticals, the health care system spends about another dollar managing the morbidity created by drug therapy[2,3] and about half the patient morbidities are preventable.[4]

MEDICAL COSTS OF DIABETES

Patients with diabetes have a great deal to lose when the drug-use process fails. Atherosclerotic cardiovascular disease and amputation increase dramatically among aging patients with diabetes.[5] Patients with diabetes have a 16-fold increased risk for lower extremity amputations compared with people who do not have diabetes[6] and a 6-fold increased risk for blindness compared to people without diabetes.[7] A 10-year follow-up of patients with diabetes in the Wisconsin Epidemiologic Study of Diabetes Retinopathy showed a high incidence of retinopathy among insulin-dependent (IDDM) and non–insulin-dependent patients with diabetes (NIDDM), with an increased incidence of proliferative diabetic retinopathy in older-onset patients whether or not they were taking insulin.[8] Patients with diabetes are also 2.3 times more likely to be hospitalized compared to age-matched people without diabetes.[7]

Intensive diabetes therapy reduces the incidence and progression of diabetic complications. The Diabetes Control and Complications Trial (DCCT), involving more than 1,400 Type I patients with diabetes at 29 North American centers, has clearly shown the benefits of improved glycemic control among IDDM patients.[9] Development and progression of long-term complications, including retinopathy, clinical neuropathy, microalbuminuria, and albuminuria, were slowed in the intensive treatment group compared to the conventional treatment group. On the other hand, the major adverse event associated with intensive therapy was a two- to three-fold increase in severe hypoglycemia. The increased hypoglycemia may be important in cognitive decline in patients with diabetes, especially among postmenopausal females.[10]

A new standard of practice is needed in the United States because current medical care for patients with diabetes neither meets the guidelines from the American Diabetes Association (ADA),[11] nor approaches the levels of care provided to the intensive treatment group in the DCCT.[12] National surveys of the level of care received by patients with diabetes indicate that only 36 percent to 65 percent of patients with diabetes see their physician at least four times yearly and that less than half the patients with diabetes see an ophthalmologist annually.[13] Furthermore, while the DCCT intensive treatment patients received extensive and frequent education, national surveys indicate only 24 percent to 59 percent of patients with diabetes have ever attended a patient education class.[13]

With respect to the current drug-use process, its major weakness occurs after the patient leaves the pharmacy with his or her diabetes medication. Many patients are left on their own to monitor their response to the drug treatment and to handle the drug-related problems that sometimes occur. Physicians and pharmacists often do not closely monitor patients' responses to drug therapy.

PHARMACEUTICAL CARE

Pharmaceutical care has been studied as a method for reducing the amount of preventable drug-related morbidity in patients with diabetes and patients with other chronic diseases. Pharmaceutical care has been defined as "the responsible provision of drug therapy for the purpose of achieving definite outcomes that improves a patient's quality-of-life."[1(p.539)] Pharmaceutical care addresses the role of health care providers in the drug-use process and may be the most critical societal purpose for the profession of pharmacy. This concept strategically redefines the drug-use process into a pharmaceutical care system in which a health professional (the pharmacist) takes responsibility for monitoring the effects of drugs and acts to resolve drug-related problems before they become a drug-related morbidity.

A pharmaceutical care system recognizes that safe and effective drug therapy requires three steps[4]:

1. preparing a therapeutic plan for a patient, including patient-specific objectives
2. dispensing a prescription along with patient education
3. monitoring of drug therapy in a system of care including patients, pharmacists, and physicians

A pharmaceutical care system assumes that more is needed to ensure good patient outcomes than prescribing a "drug of choice." In fact, the literature concerning preventable drug-related morbidity[1] suggests that much of the drug-related morbidity occurs even when the drug of choice was prescribed. Analysis of this literature suggests that the greatest weakness in the present drug-use process is that "good" drugs are monitored poorly or not at all. Pharmaceutical care represents the inclusion of "responsibility for monitoring" in the drug-use process.

The activities performed by pharmacists in providing pharmaceutical care can be conceptually classified into six major domains, including[14]:

1. documenting information
2. assessing the patient
3. establishing a therapeutic plan and a monitoring plan
4. screening a patient's record for drug-related problems
5. advising/counseling the patient
6. verifying that the patient understands his or her responsibilities

These domains represent a set of specific activities considered essential for monitoring patients' progress toward their therapeutic objectives and managing drug-related problems. Some examples of specific activities included within the aforementioned domains are (1) documenting information about the patient's medical condition, (2) asking a patient questions to assess actual patterns of medication use, and (3) asking a patient questions to find out if he or she is experiencing drug-related problems.

IMPROVING DRUG THERAPY MONITORING OF PATIENTS WITH DIABETES

Just as new standards of practice are needed in the management of patients with diabetes by physicians, a new practice standard is also in order for the pharmacist who participates in the care of patients with diabetes. One method for achieving a new practice standard is to implement a pharmaceutical care system that uses practice guidelines to help a pharmacist provide consistent care to all patients with diabetes. Pharmacists can develop a pharmaceutical care system on their own or choose to use a system developed by an organization that can be adapted for use in a particular pharmacy. One example of a pharmaceutical care system that is in use by community and clinic pharmacists is called Therapeutic Outcomes Monitoring (TOM).[4] (For further information about the Therapeutic Outcomes Monitoring program, contact the Dubow Family Center for Research in Pharmaceutical Care, University of Florida, P.O. Box 100496, Gainesville, FL 32610.)

The focus of TOM is in two general areas: (1) providing guidelines to help pharmacists monitor patients' drug therapy and (2) providing guidelines to assist pharmacists in managing drug therapy in cooperation with the patient and physician. In learning how to implement pharmaceutical care, pharmacists can choose to start with the monitoring component only by learning to recognize when a patient's disease condition is uncontrolled, when a patient is failing on his or her drug therapy, or when a patient is experiencing an adverse drug reaction. As pharmacists develop more experience, they can use the guidelines available for managing drug therapy, including steps to be taken in resolving specific types of drug-related problems.

TOM is disease based with modules available in asthma, diabetes mellitus, and several other chronic conditions. The modules provide information about most areas needed for implementing pharmaceutical care[15]:

- practice guidelines for the assessment of disease control, the identification of drug-related problems, and ways for resolving drug-related problems
- clinical record system featuring forms for patient assessment, record keeping, communications, and reporting
- brief self-study materials on the physiologic and pharmacologic basis of managing therapy in such patients
- patient education materials

- advice and information on how to obtain therapeutic data (e.g., glucose levels)
- performance-based evaluation system for use in collecting performance measures consistent with accreditation agency requirements
- description of the service for use in marketing
- advice on how to price, market, and sell TOM services
- sample offer and contract for services
- patient referral and medical necessity form with a checklist of what services are requested

Pharmacists walk through a step-by-step process as they use TOM to monitor and manage patients. For a new patient or a patient starting on his or her first medication for diabetes, the process starts with a pharmacist collecting background information about the patient's condition by using a medical patient questionnaire and interview. Pharmacists then record specific therapeutic objectives for their patients, often in cooperation with the physician providing care to the patient. Next, pharmacists assess the patient's condition with respect to the therapeutic objectives set for the patient using specific assessment parameters provided in the TOM module. Examples of data collected and then documented in the patient monitoring record include whether the patient has experienced polyuria or blurred vision since his or her last visit with the pharmacist; whether the patient has completed a foot care protocol; whether the patient's fasting plasma glucose level is >200 mg/dL, postprandial glucose level is >235 mg/dL, or glycosylated hemoglobin level is >9 percent; and whether the patient experienced an unscheduled physician visit, emergency department visit, or hospitalization since his or her last encounter with the pharmacist.

Next, the pharmacist assesses the patient's knowledge of his or her disease state and drug therapy using a set of questions provided in the TOM patient education record. Based on any knowledge gaps detected during this assessment, the pharmacist develops a patient education program customized to the patient. The patient education step is especially important in caring for patients with diabetes. Incorporation of the need for diabetes education into *Healthy People 2000*[16] acknowledges the consideration of education in reducing the morbidity and mortality of diabetes.[17] Patient education has been found to contribute to improving self-care and metabolic control of patients with diabetes.[18–20] Additionally, an improvement in a diabetic patient's perceived quality of life may also be realized through a patient education program that increases understanding and responsibility in the self-management of his or her condition.[19]

The pharmacist next assesses the patient's diabetic medications using guidelines developed for each antidiabetic medication and subsequently reviews all of the patient's other medications for possible or actual drug-related problems. Finally, the pharmacist dispenses the medication and provides patient education. This initial encounter ends with the establishment of a monitoring plan for the patient specifying when the next follow-up will occur. In some cases, the TOM guidelines advise pharmacists to follow up within a few days of dispensing a medication to see if the patient's condition is better controlled or if the patient is experiencing any problems related to the medication. Follow-ups can sometimes be handled using the telephone and in some cases will require a scheduled appointment.

These steps are the beginning of a monitoring cycle of care that never ends. Patients will often require regular assessments to help ensure that they are moving toward their therapeutic objectives. TOM provides the guidelines used for monitoring patients at each subsequent encounter between the pharmacist and the patient. When patients are experiencing poor control of their disease or a drug-related problem, specific guidelines are provided for the pharmacist. In some cases, the problem can be handled by the pharmacist as, for example, in the case where the patient is having difficulty correctly administering his or her medication. In other cases, the problem will require physician involvement. Guidelines include information that pharmacists may use in offering drug therapy recommendations to the patient's physician.

RELATIONSHIPS

Pharmaceutical care can only be provided when meaningful relationships are in place between the patient, pharmacist, and physician. Pharmacists need access to information to adequately monitor patients, and pharmacists will need to develop relationships to gain access to data. Without a collegial relationship in place between the pharmacist and physician, it is unlikely that pharmacists will have access to the data needed to monitor patients, and it is unlikely that physicians will work cooperatively in resolving patients' drug-related problems.

Despite the type of setting in which a pharmacist practices, he or she can develop collegial relationships with physicians. While pharmacists who practice in a clinic setting may have easy access to patient information, community pharmacists can also access the information they need. Community pharmacists will need to develop formal communication exchanges with physicians and their staff so that personnel in the physician's office understand why they should give the pharmacist patient information when he or she requests it.

RESOURCES FOR IMPLEMENTING PHARMACEUTICAL CARE

Implementing pharmaceutical care is not easy for pharmacists who have not placed an emphasis on monitoring patients' drug therapy in the past. Using guidelines such as those provided in the TOM modules can help a pharmacist implement pharmaceutical care, but it does not address all of the resources needed to implement and sustain a pharmaceutical care service. Other resources needed often include having a commitment by management that is supportive of pharmacists who provide pharmaceutical care, having time to care for patients, having a good information system that can track patient data, having adequate and quality space to meet with patients, and having payors who compensate pharmacists who show that they can reduce health care costs.

• • •

Drug therapy outcomes research shows that the present drug-use process could be improved. Increasing the number of pharmacists who monitor drug therapy could reduce the amount of preventable drug-related morbidity in patients with diabetes. A system such as TOM is a way for providing pharmaceutical care in ambulatory settings that emphasizes the role of the pharmacist in addressing a major cause of preventable drug-related morbidity.

REFERENCES

1. Hepler, C.D., and Strand, L.M. "Opportunities and Responsibilities in Pharmaceutical Care." *American Journal of Hospital Pharmacy* 47 (1990): 533–43.

2. Johnson, J.A., and Bootman, J.L. "Drug Related Morbidity and Mortality: A Cost-of-Illness Model." *Archives of Internal Medicine* 155 (1995): 1,949–56.

3. Lakashmanan, M.C., Hershey, C.O., and Breslau, D. "Hospital Admissions Caused by Iatrogenic Disease." *Archives of Internal Medicine* 146 (1986): 1,931–34.

4. Hepler, C.D., and Grainger-Rousseau, T.J. "Pharmaceutical Care versus Traditional Drug Treatment: Is There a Difference?" *Drugs* 49 (1995): 1–10.

5. Kannell, W.B., and McGee, D.L. "Diabetes and Cardiovascular Disease: The Framingham Study." *Journal of the American Medical Association* 241 (1979): 2,035–38.

6. Most, R.S, and Sinnock, P. "The Epidemiology of Lower Extremity Amputations in Diabetic Individuals." *Diabetes Care* 6 (1983): 87–91.

7. National Society to Prevent Blindness. *Vision Problems in the U.S.* New York: 1980.

8. Klein, R., et al. "The Wisconsin Epidemiologic Study of Diabetic Retinopathy: XIV. Ten-Year Incidence and Progression of Diabetic Retinopathy." *Archives of Ophthalmology* 112 (1994): 1,217–28.

9. Diabetes Control and Complications Trial (DCCT) Research Group. "The Effect of Intensive Treatment of Diabetes on the Development and Progression of Long-

Term Complications in Insulin-Dependent Diabetes Mellitus." *New England Journal of Medicine* 329, no. 14 (1993): 977–86.

10. Rajakumar, G., deFibre, N., and Simpkins, N. "Estradiol Reduces Cognitive Decline Caused by Severe Hypoglycemia." (Paper presented at the annual meeting of the Society for Neuroscience, San Diego, CA, November 11–16, 1995).

11. American Diabetes Association. "Standards of Medical Care for Patients with Diabetes Mellitus." *Diabetes Care* 17 (1994): 616–23.

12. Tuttleman, M., Lipsett, L., and Harris, M.I. "Attitudes and Behaviors of Primary Care Physicians Regarding Tight Control of Blood Glucose in IDDM Patients." *Diabetes Care* 16 (1993): 765–72.

13. Harris, M.I., Eastman, R.C., and Siebert, C. "The DCCT and Medical Care for Diabetics in the U.S." *Diabetes Care* 17 (1994): 761–64.

14. Odedina, F., and Segal, R. "Behavioral Pharmaceutical Care Scale for Measuring Pharmacists' Activities." *American Journal of Health-System Pharmacists* 53 (1996): 855–65.

15. Grainger-Rousseau, T.J., et al. "Therapeutic Outcomes Monitoring: Monitoring and Managing Patient Outcomes in Community Pharmacy." (In review).

16. Department of Health and Human Services. *Healthy People 2000: National Health Promotion and Disease Prevention Objectives.* DHHS publ. No. PHS 91-50212. Washington, DC: U.S. Government Printing Office, 1991.

17. Coonrod, B.A., Betschart, J., and Harris, M.I. "Frequency and Determinants of Diabetes Patient Education Among Adults in the U.S. Population." *Diabetes Care* 17 (1994): 852–58.

18. Mazzuca, S.A., et al. "The Diabetes Education Study: A Controlled Trial of the Effects of Diabetes Patient Education." *Diabetes Care* 9 (1986): 1–10.

19. Rubin, R.R., Peyrot, M., and Saudek, C.D. "Effect of Diabetes Education on Self-Care, Metabolic Control, and Emotional Well-Being." *Diabetes Care* 12 (1989): 673–79.

20. Peyrot, M., and Rubin, R.R. "Modeling the Effect of Diabetes Education on Glycemic Control." *Diabetes Educator* 13 (1987): 206–09.

PART II

Drug Therapy of Type II Diabetes Mellitus

Oral hypoglycemic agents have been the cornerstone of therapy for the treatment of type II diabetes mellitus. They allow patients to avoid insulin injections and, when combined with diet and exercise, offer excellent treatment success. The authors of the chapters in this section focus on the use of drugs in the treatment of diabetes. Sulfonylureas continue to be useful in treatment and find new roles and enhanced success when combined with new agents. The recent past has seen the release of a number of new agents in the United States. The roles of these agents will be fully defined in the patient care arena; however, several offer clear improvements and changes in outcomes. No drug comes without the cost of adverse reactions and therapeutic misadventures; this aspect of therapy selection and monitoring is also emphasized. All three chapters in this section highlight the opportunities from currently available drugs and forecast areas where research may provide additional therapeutic alternatives.

CHAPTER 6

Exploring the Role of Sulfonylureas in the Treatment of Non–Insulin-Dependent Diabetes Mellitus

John P. Graham, PharmD and Darren M. Stam, PharmD

For the last 30 years, sulfonylureas have been the mainstay of treatment for patients with non–insulin-dependent diabetes mellitus (NIDDM). They offered patients an alternative to using insulin to lower their blood glucose. One of the advantages of these agents was that they could be taken orally as opposed to insulin, which required multiple daily injections. In addition, they are tolerable, with few side effects, and they cause less hypoglycemia than does insulin. In the past year, new agents (metformin and acarbose) have been introduced into the market and have offered practitioners an alternative to the traditional sulfonylureas. The sulfonylureas are still valuable agents in the treatment of NIDDM. Their efficacy is unsurpassed by any other oral medications. They possess the best tolerability profile of all oral agents on the market, and they possess very few contraindications or drug interactions. The sulfonylureas should still be considered first-line agents for NIDDM. Metformin and acarbose are agents that may benefit a specific patient population, but sulfonylureas are agents that can benefit most patients. Key words: *adverse effects, hyperglycemia, macrovascular disease, NIDDM, pharmacology, sulfonylureas, Type II Diabetes*

INTRODUCTION

In recent years, the importance in intensive treatment of diabetes mellitus has been highlighted with the publication of the Diabetes Control and Complications Trial (DCCT). The DCCT concluded that intensive control of insulin-dependent diabetes mellitus (IDDM) could greatly reduce the incidence of microvascular complications that have always been associated with diabetes.[1] These complications, which include retinopathy, nephropathy, and neuropathies, contribute to the significant disabilities and the significant costs associated with diabetes.[1] Smaller studies have also highlighted the importance of intensive treatment with oral medications and insulin in the treatment of non–insulin-dependent diabetes mellitus (NIDDM).[2,3]

NIDDM patients comprise greater than 90 percent of all patients with diabetes mellitus.[4,5] Traditionally, patients with NIDDM were controlled on diet first, then, as diet failed to keep blood sugars low enough, sulfonylureas were used as the primary pharmacologic therapy. Once the patient's diabetes progressed enough that sulfonylureas were not controlling the blood glucose, the patient either had to have insulin added to the sulfonylurea or be completely switched to insulin. In reaction to the lack of available therapies, and in response to the growing number of patients with NIDDM, the pharmaceutical industry has developed new oral medications to combat the hyperglycemia associated with NIDDM. Two of the current medications available, metformin and acarbose, have been widely accepted as alternatives to sulfonylureas. The significant differences in mechanisms between these two agents and sulfonylureas have promoted debate over which medication should be used in specific situations and whether sulfonylureas should still be considered the initial medication of choice. This article will answer these and other common questions about sulfonylureas by comparing and contrasting the mechanism of action of sulfonylureas to the newer agents and then defining the role of sulfonylureas in the treatment of NIDDM.

PATHOPHYSIOLOGY OF NIDDM

In order to understand the role of a particular medication in a disease state, it is important to understand the relationship between the pathogenesis of the disease and the mechanism of medication. In addition, it is important to understand the relationships between the available medications, their respective mechanisms of actions, and the pathogenesis of NIDDM.

NIDDM is a result of an apparent lack of insulin. This apparent lack of insulin results from two mechanisms: (1) a decreased insulin release in response to a glucose load and (2) tissue resistance to the effects of insulin. Due to the impaired insulin response and tissue resistance, the cells of the body will experience a lack of intracellular glucose. In response to this cellular hypoglycemia, the body will respond by increasing the hepatic production of glucose, also known as *glucoeogenesis,* and by stimulating the appetite centers to increase the consumption of carbohydrates. In response, the body may increase the production of insulin, resulting in hyperinsulinemia.[6-11] The understanding of these different pathogenic mechanisms will allow the medical community to treat NIDDM with a combination of medications, which, because of their diverse mechanisms of action, will result in significantly lower blood sugar.

Two new medications, metformin and acarbose, have given diabetes practitioners alternatives to the more traditional regimens of sulfonylureas or insulin in patients with NIDDM. In contrast to sulfonylureas and exogenous insulin,

the newer agents have been designed to decrease fasting blood glucose, postprandial glucose, and glycosylated hemoglobin without increasing insulin and, therefore, avoiding the possible cardiovascular effects of hyperinsulinemia and the detrimental effects of weight gain.[6-19]

METFORMIN

Metformin, the only biguanide available, does not stimulate insulin secretion but lowers serum glucose by inhibiting glucose production, increasing the sensitivity of peripheral tissues to the effect of insulin, and decreasing the absorption of glucose in the stomach. The result of these multiple mechanisms is a decrease in fasting blood glucose and a significant reduction in glycosylated hemoglobin.[19-29] Metformin has been shown in a number of studies to reduce the HbA_{1c} by as much as 1 to 2 percent.[19-29,34] In addition, metformin has been used in patients who are already on insulin to decrease the amount of insulin required. One of the most important aspects of metformin is that while it has a significant effect on HbA_{1c} and fasting blood glucose, it does not increase insulin levels. Patients with lowered or unaffected insulin levels do not experience the typical increase in appetite and weight associated with insulin and sulfonylureas. As a result, in patients in whom increased weight could be detrimental, metformin may be the alternative of choice.[19-29]

On the negative side, metformin is associated with less tolerability than sulfonylureas. The most severe and important side effect of metformin is lactic acidosis. Lactic acidosis occurs in less than 0.01 to 0.08 cases per 1,000 patient years; however, in patients who develop lactic acidosis, the mortality rate approaches 50 percent. Most of the cases of lactic acidosis can be attributed to its use in patients who exhibit contraindications to the medication. These include patients with renal insufficiency, liver dysfunction, decreased tissue perfusion (i.e., severe infection with hypotension), or alcohol abuse and patients receiving radiographic contrast agents. Additional adverse effects consist primarily of gastrointestinal symptoms (diarrhea, nausea, vomiting, flatulence, anorexia), metallic taste, and impaired absorption of vitamin B12.[19-29]

ACARBOSE

The alpha-glucosidase inhibitor acarbose decreases serum blood sugar by inhibiting the enzyme that breaks down carbohydrates in the small intestine. The inhibition of alpha-glucosidase results in a delay in carbohydrate absorption, therefore decreasing postprandial blood glucose and subsequently fasting blood glucose. As with metformin, acarbose does not stimulate insulin secretion; therefore, either a decrease or no change in the patient's weight results. This again could be beneficial in patients with comorbid conditions that may be exacerbated by an increase in weight.[28-34]

Adverse effects of acarbose include significant gastrointestinal symptoms in up to 30 percent of patients. These effects include nausea, vomiting, diarrhea, flatulence, and bloating. Smaller studies have shown that these effects subside after a short duration of therapy. These effects can also be minimized by decreasing the amount of carbohydrates that a person consumes with each meal. Acarbose is not significantly absorbed into the circulation, so the systemic effects are minimal, with a rare increase in liver transaminase levels.[28-34]

SULFONYLUREAS

Mechanism of Action

Since the development of sulfonylureas in the 1950s, it has been postulated that they have multiple mechanisms of action. These proposed mechanisms include stimulation of insulin release, inhibition of hepatic glucose production, and sensitization of peripheral tissues to insulin. These mechanisms can be divided into two sections: pancreatic and extrapancreatic effects.[35-53]

Pancreatic Effects

One of the tissue abnormalities associated with NIDDM includes the defective secretion of insulin by the pancreas. Traditionally, sulfonylureas' ability to lower blood glucose was attributed to their ability to stimulate the production and secretion of insulin from the pancreas. This mechanism is not fully understood but involves the stimulation of beta cells in the pancreas, which are responsible for insulin production and secretion. This effect has been proven through multiple studies, which have shown an increase in insulin levels both in response to a glucose challenge and in fasting states. Although the response to sulfonylureas is independent of glucose levels, the pancreatic response will be larger in patients with higher serum glucose levels. This phenomenon is not completely understood, but it is thought that the response of the beta-cells to sulfonylureas and glucose is additive in patients with elevated glucose levels. For example, a patient with lower serum glucose levels would continue to have the insulin stimulation from the sulfonylurea but not the stimulation from glucose. In contrast, in a patient with higher serum glucose, the pancreas will be stimulated by both the sulfonylurea and the elevated glucose level.[7,35-41,45,46]

Further proof of this mechanism comes from the failure of sulfonylureas to be efficacious in patients with IDDM. These patients lack pancreatic function, therefore rendering any medication that would stimulate insulin production worthless.

Extrapancreatic Effects

Over the years, researchers have been studying the response of the pancreas to treatment with sulfonylureas. These studies have shown a significant increase in insulin levels within the first 2 weeks of treatment, and then the levels subside back to pretreatment levels.[7,35-41,45,46] In response to this, it was proposed that sulfonylureas are exerting additional effects on areas of the body other than the pancreas.

These alternative mechanisms include the inhibition of hepatic gluconeogenesis and an increase in insulin sensitivity. Studies have shown that sulfonylureas lower the production of glucose by the liver. These studies, however, were not able to separate the effects of lowering glucose from any direct effect that sulfonylureas might have in gluconeogenesis. In patients with insulin insensitivity and hyperglycemia, the liver is stimulated to produce more glucose in response to the apparent lack of glucose and energy within the cells. Therefore, when a medication lowers the glucose levels, be it by supplying more insulin or by increasing glucose utilization, the liver will respond by decreasing the production of glucose. In addition to this explanation, sulfonylureas have been shown to be ineffective in the treatment of IDDM, which illustrates the need for a functioning pancreas in patients using sulfonylureas.

Smaller studies have shown increased sensitivity of tissues to insulin after treatment with insulin, but they have not developed a mechanism for this phenomenon. The concept of insulin sensitization is not completely understood, but it is thought to be involved in reducing plasma glucose. However, we cannot estimate the degree to which this mechanism contributes to the overall reduction.

Differences between Agents

Although there are no known differences between any sulfonylureas as far as their mechanism of action, there are differences in certain pharmacokinetic parameters, potency, and adverse reaction profiles. A complete list of available sulfonylureas with characteristics can be found in Table 1. Second generation agents are typically known to be more potent. This is not because of greater serum glucose reduction but because of equal glucose reductions using milligram doses instead of grams. Many studies have looked at the efficacy of sulfonylureas and attempted to find differences in glucose-lowering effects between agents. Studies that have compared specific agents have found comparable blood glucose reductions and similar reductions in HbA1c. Preliminary results from the United Kingdom Prospective Diabetes Study (UKPDS) at three years showed a reduction in fasting plasma glucose from baseline of approximately 14 mg/dL with glyburide and 21 mg/dL with chlorpropamide. The levels compared to placebo were reduced 36 mg/dL and 28.8 mg/dL for chlorpropamide and glyburide respectively. The HbA1c during the same three years, when compared to placebo, was 0.8 percent lower for chlorpropamide and 0.7 percent lower for glyburide.[32] Other studies have shown reductions from 0.5 to 2 percent mostly depending on the baseline HbA1c.[7,30–32,50,51] The larger end of the scale was in studies with higher baseline HbA1c.

The first generation agents range from short acting (tolbutamide), requiring twice-daily doses, to longer acting (chlorpropamide), which

Table 1. Sulfonylureas available

Compounds	Generic name	Brand name	Dosage range (mg.)	Dosage regimen	Duration of action (hr.)	Onset of action
First generation	Tolbutamide	Orinase	500–3,000	bid	6–10	Fast
	Chlorpropamide	Diabinese	100–750	qd	48–60	Slow
	Acetohexamide	Dymelor	250–1,500	qd-bid	12–18	Fast
	Tolazamide	Tolinase	100–1,000	qd-bid	12–24	Medium
Second generation	Glyburide	Diabeta Micronase	2.5–20	qd-bid	20–24	Medium
		Glynase	3.5–12	qd-bid	14–16	
	Glipazide	Glucotrol	2.4–40	qd-bid	10–15	Fast
		Glucotrol XL	5–20	qd	24	Medium
	Glimepiride	Amaryl	1–8	qd	24	Fast

has a duration of activity of up to 60 hours.[7,38] Second generation agents have also been associated with higher rates of adverse effects. These effects include an increased risk of hypoglycemia with longer acting agents and an increased risk of experiencing hematologic, dermatologic, and endocrinology side effects. Due to these differences, it is recommended that new onset NIDDM patients be initiated on a second generation agent. Patients who have been controlled on first generation agents without problems do not need to be changed to a second generation agent.

With the recent addition of glimepiride to the second generation sulfonylureas, the argument over differences between agents within classes has resurfaced. In small animal studies, glimepiride exhibited an insulin-sparing effect that stimulated some conversation about it actually being a third generation agent. This insulin-sparing effect has not been exhibited in human trials, and, at this time, it is still classified as second generation.[37,39,49] Throughout the years, the medical community has tried to define differences between glyburide and glipazide. Glyburide has a much longer duration of activity, which has been associated with a greater risk of hypoglycemia. The two agents have shown similar reductions in fasting blood glucose and HbA1c. All sulfonylureas have reduced HbA1c by up to 1 to 2 percent with no differences found between agents.[7,32,40,50]

Sulfonylureas have typically been known as one of the most tolerable classes of medications. The overall incidence of adverse effects with all sulfonylureas is reported to be approximately 3 to 4 percent. Chlorpropamide has been associated with the greatest incidence of adverse effects, which is reported at 4.1 percent. The most common adverse effects are gastrointestinal (nausea, vomiting, dyspepsia) and dermatologic (pruritis, erythema). Elevations in liver transaminase levels are rare but possible. These elevations are less frequent with second generation than with first, probably due to the need for less medication to produce the same glucose-lowering effects. The incidence of hypoglyce-

mia with sulfonylureas is common, with the Swedish Adverse Reaction Registry showing a rate of 0.22 episodes per 1,000 patient years. This, however, is much lower than the rate seen with insulin, which is approximately 100 episodes per 1,000 patient years.[7,38] Agents with longer durations of action, such as chlorpropamide and glyburide, are associated with a higher incidence of hypoglycemia.[7,38]

One of the more controversial issues regarding the use of sulfonylureas is the possible risk of macrovascular disease associated with increased levels of insulin. In the late 1960s, the University Group Diabetes Program, a multi-centered trial, was discontinued early because there was a significant increase in cardiovascular mortality in patients taking tolbutamide or phenformin when compared to those patients treated with diet alone. This study has been one of the most debated studies of all time and continues to be used as an example of poorly designed studies. Even with this criticism, the Food and Drug Administration (FDA) has continued to require a warning be placed in the package inserts of all sulfonylureas and all biguanides.[52] Until recently, practitioners did not put much stock in the results from this trial and have not hesitated in the use of sulfonylureas. The recent publication of the results from the Quebec Cardiovascular Study, implicating hyperinsulinemia as an independent risk factor for macrovascular disease, has stimulated new discussions on the implications of sulfonylureas in development of macrovascular disease. The study was performed in healthy, nondiabetic men 45 to 76 years of age who had no history of ischemic heart disease. The odds ratio for ischemic heart disease in patients with hyperinsulinemia was 1.7 (95 percent confidence interval; 1.3 to 2.4). After adjustment for known risk factors for ischemic heart disease, the odds ratio was 1.6 (95 percent confidence interval; 1.1 to 2.3). The major limitation of this study involves the use of healthy, nondiabetic males, therefore rendering these results inconclusive for diabetic patients.[18] Results from the Paris Prospective Study and the Helsinki Study failed to implicate hyperinsulinemia as an independent risk factor.[13,17-19,53] They showed an increased relationship between insulin levels, but, when other factors such as high-density lipoprotein (HDL) cholesterol were taken into account, the independent association was not significant.

The controversy that these studies illustrate is a vital issue in deciding the role of sulfonylureas in NIDDM. If a relationship exists between hyperinsulinemia and macrovascular disease, and if this is shown to be true in diabetic patients, then sulfonylureas will not be the agent of choice in many patients. The UKPDS trial, an ongoing trial comparing sulfonylureas, insulin, and metformin, will help to answer this question by determining whether glycemic control will prevent diabetic complications and whether one agent will decrease or increase mortality or morbidity greater than another.[32] Until the results of this trial are published, there will not be an answer to the question of whether there is a link between sulfonylureas and macrovascular complications, and we must for now conclude that they are still beneficial agents for most NIDDM patients.

•   •   •

In recent years, new oral diabetic medications, new insulin products, and large studies have revolutionized the treatment of diabetes mellitus. In a time of change, it is easy to ignore older therapies that still have value and may still be the agents of choice. This may be happening to sulfonylureas. Newer drugs give a practitioner an option for treating NIDDM with a different mechanism of action, but they have not shown they are more effective than sulfonylureas. They also have limitations to their use, which include contraindications and adverse reactions.

Sulfonylureas are effective, tolerable agents for the treatment of NIDDM. They have proven over the years to reduce plasma glucose levels and HbA1c, and investigators will soon be able to evaluate whether they reduce complications associated with NIDDM. The DCCT left the medical community with proof that intensive treatment of IDDM can significantly reduce the incidence of diabetic complications, and the UKPDS should be able to answer these questions in NIDDM patients.

Sulfonylureas are still the mainstay of treatment in NIDDM. They are as effective as any other treatment, and they are more tolerable than other oral medications. As the American Diabetes Association stated in their Consensus Statement on the Pharmacologic Treatment of Patients with NIDDM, "Sulfonylureas are a rational choice to begin pharmacologic intervention because almost all patients with NIDDM are relatively insulin deficient."[26(p.S56)]

REFERENCES

1. The Diabetes Control and Complications Trial Research Group, "The Effect of Intensive Treatment of Diabetes on the Development and Progression of Long-term Complications in Insulin-dependent Diabetes Mellitus," *New England Journal of Medicine* 329, no. 14 (1993): 977–986.

2. R.R. Henry et al., "Intensive Conventional Insulin Therapy for Type II Diabetes: Metabolic Effects During a 6-month Outpatient Trial." *Diabetes Care* 17 (1993): 21–31.

3. R. Klein et al., "Glycosylated Hemoglobin Predicts the Incidence and Progression of Diabetic Retinopathy," *JAMA* 260 (1988): 2,864–2,871.

4. "CDC Surveillance for Diabetes Mellitus—United States," *Morbidity and Mortality Weekly Report* 42, no. 1 (1980–1989).

5. American Diabetes Association, *Diabetes 1993 Vital Statistics* (Alexandria, VA: 1993).

6. D.M. Nathan, "The Pathophysiology of Diabetic Complications: How Much Does Glucose Hypothesis Explain?" *Annals of Internal Medicine* 124 (1996): 86–89.

7. L.C. Groop, "Sulfonylureas in NIDDM," *Diabetes Care* 15, no. 6 (1992): 737–751.

8. P.J. Campbell et al., "Quantification of the Relative Impairment in Actions of Insulin on Hepatic Glucose Production and Peripheral Glucose Uptake in Non–insulin-dependent Diabetes Mellitus," *Metabolism* 37 (1988): 15–21.

9. T.W. Garvey et al., "The Effect of Insulin Treatment on Insulin Secretion and Insulin Action in Type II Diabetes Mellitus." *Diabetes* 34 (1985): 222–234.

10. W.J. Andrews et al., "Insulin Therapy in Obese, Non-Insulin Dependent Diabetes Induces Improvements in Insulin Action and Secretion that Are Maintained for Two Weeks after Insulin Withdrawal," *Diabetes* 33 (1984): 634–642.

11. R. Klein et al., "Relation of Glycemic Control to Diabetic Microvascular Complications in Diabetes Mellitus." *Annals of Internal Medicine,* 124 (1996): 90–96.

12. R. Klein, "Hyperglycemia and Microvascular and Macrovascular Disease in Diabetes," *Diabetes Care* 18, no. 2 (1995): 258–268.

13. H. Kleen, "Insulin Resistance and the Prevention of Diabetes Mellitus." *New England Journal of Medicine* 331, no. 18 (1994): 1,226–1,227.

14. M.I. Harris, "Undiagnosed NIDDM: Clinical and Public Health Issues," *Diabetes Care* 16 (1993): 977–986.

15. G.M. Reaven, "Role of Insulin Resistance in Human Disease." *Diabetes* 37 (1988): 1,595–1,607.

16. G. Pogatsa, "Potassium Channels in the Cardiovascular System," *Diabetes Research and Clinical Practice* 28, suppl. (1995): S91–S98.

17. P. McKeigue, and G. Davey, "Associations between Insulin Levels and Cardiovascular Disease are Confounded by Comorbidity," *Diabetes Care* 18, no. 9 (1995): 1,294–1,298.

18. J. Despres et al., "Hyperinsulinemia as an Independent Risk Factor for Ischemic Heart Disease." *New England Journal of Medicine* 334, no. 15 (1996): 952–956.

19. E. Grossman, F.H. Messerli, "Diabetic Hypertensive Heart Disease," *Annals of Internal Medicine* 125 (1996): 304–310.

20. C.J. Bailey, "Biguanides and NIDDM," *Diabetes Care* 15, no. 6 (1992): 755–772.

21. D. Giugliano et al., "Metformin for Obese, Insulin-treated Diabetic Patients: Improvement in Glycemic Control and Reduction of Metabolic Risk Factors." *European Journal of Clinical Pharmacology* 44 (1993): 107–112.

22. C.J. Bailey et al., "Metformin." *New England Journal of Medicine* 334, no. 9 (1996): 574–579.

23. L.D. Hermann et al., "Therapeutic Comparison of Metformin and Sulfonylureas, Alone and in Combinations," *Diabetes Care* 17, no. 10 (1994): 1,100–1,109.

24. G. Perriello et al., "Acute Antihyperglycemic Mechanism of Metformin in NIDDM: Evidence for Suppression of Lipid Oxidation and Hepatic Glucose Production," *Diabetes* 43 (1994): 920–928.

25. Z.T. Bloomgarden, "New and Traditional Treatment of Glycemia in NIDDM," *Diabetes Care* 19, no. 3 (1996): 295–299.

26. American Diabetes Association, "Consensus Statement: "The Pharmacologic Treatment of Hyperglycemia in NIDDM," *Diabetes Care* 19, no. 1 (1996): s54–s61.

27. J. Chiasson et al., "The Efficacy of Acarbose in the Treatment of Patients with Non-insulin-dependent Diabetes Mellitus," *Annals of Internal Medicine* 121, no. 12 (1994): 928–935.

28. R.R. Coniff et al., "Reduction of Glycosylated Hemoglobin and Postprandial Hyperglycemia by Acarbose in Patients with NIDDM," *Diabetes Care* 18, no. 6 (1995): 817–823.

29. R.R. Coniff et al., "A Double-blind Placebo Controlled Trial Evaluating the Safety and Efficacy of Acarbose for the Treatment of Patients with Insulin-requiring Type II Diabetes," *Diabetes Care* 18, no. 7 (1995): 928–932.

30. J. Hommfann, and M. Spengler, "Efficacy of 24-week Monotherapy with Acarbose, Glibenclamide, or Placebo in NIDDM Patients," *Diabetes Care* 17, no. 6 (1994): 561–565.

31. R.R. Coniff et al., "Multicenter, Placebo-controlled Trial Comparing Acarbose (BAY g 5421) with Placebo, Tolbutamide, and Tolbutamide-plus-acarbose in Non-insulin-dependent Diabetes Mellitus," *American Journal of Medicine* 98 (1995): 443–451.

32. United Kingdom Prospective Diabetes Study Group, "United Kingdom Prospective Diabetes Study (UKPDS) 13: Relative Efficacy of Randomly Allocated Diet, Sulphonylurea, Insulin, or Metformin in Patients with Newly Diagnosed Non-insulin Dependent Diabetes Followed for Three Years," *British Medical Journal* 310 (1995): 83–88.

33. B.F. Clarke, and I.W. Campbell, "Comparison of Metformin and Chlorpropamide in Non-obese, Maturity-onset Diabetics Uncontrolled by Diet," *British Medical Journal* 2 (1977): 1,576–1,578.

34. M. Nattrass, and K.G.M.M. Alberti, "Biguanides," *Diabetologia* 14 (1978): 71–74.

35. T.W. Garvey et al., "The Effect of Insulin Treatment on Insulin Secretion and Insulin Action in Type II Diabetes Mellitus," *Diabetes* 34 (1985): 222–234.

36. W. J. Andrews et al., "Insulin Therapy in Obese, Non-insulin Dependent Diabetes Induces Improvements in Insulin Action and Secretion that Are Maintained for Two Weeks after Insulin Withdrawal," *Diabetes* 33 (1984): 634–642.

37. "Glimepiride for NIDDM," *The Medical Letter* 38, no. 975 (1996): 47–48.

38. M.N. Feinglos, and H.E. Lebovitz, "Sulfonylurea Treatment of Insulin-independent Diabetes Mellitus," *Metabolism* 29, no. 5 (1980): 488–494.

39. E. Draeger, "Clinical Profile of Glimepiride," *Diabetes Research and Clinical Practice* 28, suppl. (1995): S139–S146.

40. B.D. Prendergast, "Drug Reviews: Glyburide and Glipizide, Second Generation Oral Sulfonylurea Hypoglycemic Agents," *Clinical Pharmacokinetics* 3 (1984): 473–485.

41. J.F. Caro, "Effects of Glyburide on Carbohydrate Metabolism and Insulin Action in the Liver," *American Journal of Medicine* 89, suppl. 2A (1990): 17S–25S.

42. O.P. McGuinness, and A.D. Cherrington, "Effect of Glyburide on Hepatic Glucose Metabolism, *American Journal of Medicine* 89, suppl. 2A (1990): 26S–37S.

43. R.J. Smith, "Effects of the Sulfonylureas on Muscle Glucose Homeostasis," *American Journal of Medicine* 89, suppl. 2A (1990): 38S–43S.

44. D.C. Simonson, "Effects of Glyburide in In Vivo Insulin-mediated Glucose Disposal, *American Journal of Medicine* 89, suppl. 2A (1990): 44S–50S.

45. A.E. Boyd et al., "Molecular Mechanism of Action of Glyburide in the Beta Cell, *American Journal of Medicine* 89, suppl. 2A (1990): 3S–10S.

46. J.R. Gavin, "Glyburide: New Insights into Its Effects on Beta Cell and Beyond: Introduction." *American Journal of Medicine* 89, suppl. 2A (1990): 1S–2S.

47. K. Kaku et al., "Extrapancreatic Effects of Sulfonylurea Drugs," *Diabetes Research and Clinical Practice* 28, suppl. (1995): S105–S108.

48. N.M. O'Meara et al., "Effect of Glyburide on Beta Cell Responsiveness to Glucose in Non-insulin-dependent Diabetes Mellitus, *American Journal of Medicine* 89, suppl. 2A (1990): 11S–16S.

49. R. Kawamori et al., "Influence of Oral Sulfonylurea Agents in Hepatic Glucose Uptake," *Diabetes Research and Clinical Practice* 28, suppl. (1995): S109–S113.

50. M. Berelowitz et al., "Comparative Efficacy of Once-daily Controlled-release Formulation of Glipizide and Immediate-release Glipizide in Patients with NIDDM," *Diabetes Care* 17, no. 12 (1994): 1,460–1,464.

51. P.R. Prosser et al., "The 24-hour Effects of Glyburide and Chlorpropamide after Chronic Treatment of Type II Diabetic Patients," *American Journal of Sciences* 289, no. 5 (1985): 179–185.

52. The University Group Diabetic Program, "Effects of Hypoglycemic Agents on Vascular Complication in Patients with Adult-onset Diabetes. VII. Evaluation of Insulin Therapy: Final Report," *Diabetes* 31, suppl. 5 (1982): 1–26.

53. E. Eschwege et al., "Coronary Heart Disease Incidence and Cardiovascular Mortality in Relation with Diabetes, Blood Glucose and Plasma Insulin Levels: The Paris Prospective Study, Ten Years Later," *Hormone and Metabolic Research* 171, suppl. (1994): 293–296.

CHAPTER 7

New Therapeutic Options in the Treatment of Diabetes Mellitus

Cheryl Kentch Miller, PharmD

Although a number of compounds exist for the treatment of diabetes mellitus, euglycemia in many patients is still difficult or impossible to achieve. Many patients are insulin resistant, a condition that is not adequately remedied either by sulfonylureas or insulin, and usually worsens over time. In addition, there are patients that, although their fasting blood glucose is controlled, experience unacceptable postprandial glucose excursions. The newer compounds that are either approved or under development possess more novel mechanisms of action that may contribute to their efficacy in these patients. The agents reviewed in this article include those that attenuate postprandial glucose elevations by mechanisms such as delayed gastric emptying and enzyme inhibition, and those that directly increase insulin sensitivity. Key words: *alpha-glucosidase inhibitors, hypoglycemic agents, human amylin analog, insulin-like growth factors, thiazolidinediones, Type 2 diabetes mellitus*

Achieving and maintaining glucose control in patients with diabetes mellitus is a constant challenge for health care professionals. Currently, there are many therapeutic agents that can be used either as single agents or in combination to treat patients with diabetes. Despite adequate patient compliance with diet and medications, optimal glycemic control is not always achieved. In a continued search for ways of controlling diabetes mellitus, a number of agents with novel mechanisms that represent new approaches are currently being developed for market in this country. Although some are members of the same drug categories as relatively new existing drugs, most all of them are agents with novel mechanisms of action and, therefore, should be of interest to both the challenged practitioner and the patient.

While the approach to diagnosing and treating patients with diabetes mellitus is constantly evolving, the marker for assessing glycemic control is still fasting blood glucose levels. Indeed, the goal in most patients with diabetes is to maintain the fasting blood glucose as close to normal as possible while avoiding dangerous hypoglycemic episodes. Evidence exists that shows an advantage of tight glycemic control in patients with Type I diabetes or insulin-dependent diabetes mellitus (IDDM).[1] Other studies have found the same advantages for tight control in patients with Type II diabetes or non–insulin-dependent diabetes mellitus (NIDDM) as well.[2]

Development of new therapeutic modalities has been hastened in part by an increased understanding of the pathophysiology of diabetes mellitus. In healthy individuals, insulin is secreted by the beta-cells of the pancreas in response to a meal or carbohydrate load. Insulin interacts with insulin receptors and facilitates the entry of glucose into the cell where it is used for energy. The primary defect in patients with IDDM is an absence of circulating insulin, usually due to destruction of pancreatic beta cells. In contrast, NIDDM is usually characterized by either an inadequate amount of insulin secretion or a relative insulin resistance or insensitivity.[3] As the insensitivity to insulin becomes more prominent, the beta cells secrete an increasing amount of insulin to compensate for this resistance. Eventually, the beta cells are exhausted and hyperglycemia results.[3]

The current approach to patients with IDDM is diet modification, exercise, and insulin therapy. For patients with NIDDM, the more modern method of treatment has been to optimize diet therapy and weight control. However, when patients are noncompliant with these interventions or when behavior and lifestyle modifications fail, oral medications are generally the next step in therapy. Sulfonylureas have been available in this country for over 10 years. Although they are effective in lowering plasma glucose, their mechanism of action is one of increasing insulin secretion. This stimulation continues sometimes despite low blood glucose, and hypoglycemia may occur. These drugs are also relatively ineffective in patients with NIDDM without adequate insulin stores. Recently, other oral agents have been approved in the United States for treating patients with NIDDM. Acarbose is a representative of the most recent class of hypoglycemic agent to be approved for general use. Acarbose is a disaccharidase inhibitor that delays the absorption of carbohydrates, which leads to an attenuated rise in postprandial glucose.[4] However, because acarbose sets up essentially a "malabsorptive syndrome" by inhibiting absorption of nutrients, the incidence of gastrointestinal side effects is often high.[4]

Clearly, the existing therapeutic options for NIDDM are not always effective or desirable in all patients. As a result, the development of agents with alternative mechanisms of action and side-effect profiles has increased. Not only are novel agents that act by primarily decreasing blood glucose levels being developed but also agents that increase the availability and release of other hormones secreted by the beta cells of the pancreas. This review will discuss some of the newer therapies and their potential role in the therapeutic treatment of patients with diabetes.

AGENTS THAT ATTENUATE POSTPRANDIAL GLUCOSE ELEVATIONS

As mentioned previously, the primary measurement of glycemic control is fasting blood glucose levels. However, in both IDDM and NIDDM, even with controlled fasting blood glucose levels, postprandial excursions may be problematic and more difficult to control. New therapeutic agents under development include those that assist in controlling these potentially wide swings in blood glucose either by delaying gastric emptying or by blocking the absorption of complex carbohydrates.

DELAYED GASTRIC EMPTYING

Pramlintide

Insulin is secreted by the beta-cells in response to nutrient intake and acts by regulating the rate of glucose uptake and disposal. Exogenous insulin has been used for many years in the treatment of both IDDM and NIDDM. However, other hormones from the pancreatic cells also play a role in maintaining euglycemia. Glucagon, which is secreted by the alpha-cells of the pancreas, protects against hypoglycemia by stimulating hepatic glycogenolysis and gluconeogenesis in the fasting state.[5] In addition, amylin, which is cosecreted with insulin from the beta-cell, appears to be responsible for the regulation of carbohydrate uptake by delaying gastric emptying.[5] Both amylin and insulin play a role in the regulation of glycemic control by acting to suppress glucagon secretion. In a euglycemic hyperinsulinemic glucose clamp study with rats, peak glucagon levels were decreased by as much as 67 percent when given doses of amylin close to those normally circulating in rats.[6] In IDDM, beta-cell destruction results in the loss of amylin secretion, which leads to episodes of postprandial hyperglycemia that have been attributed to an increase in hepatic glucose production.[7] This increase may be caused by a lack of suppression of endogenous glucagon. With NIDDM, beta-cell exhaustion often occurs, which results in a decrease in amylin secretion. This results in excessive hepatic glucagon production due to lack of suppression of plasma glucagon postprandially.

Gastric emptying times for patients with IDDM and NIDDM are accelerated as compared with healthy individuals.[8] Therefore, patients with IDDM and NIDDM often show a more rapid appearance of glucose in the blood stream following a meal than do healthy individuals. Delay of gastric emptying is a way of regulating the rate at which oral nutrients enter the systemic circulation.[9] This delay has been associated with a decrease in the postprandial hyperglycemia often seen in patients with IDDM and NIDDM.[9]

Human amylin is a 37-amino acid peptide hormone.[10] A tripro-amylin analog of this compound, pramlintide (AC137; Amylin Pharmaceuticals), is currently in development as adjunct therapy to insulin in the treatment of patients with IDDM and NIDDM.[9] Studies in diabetic rats demonstrated a dose-dependent suppression of gastric emptying with amylin concentrations considered within physiologic concentrations for this animal.[11] In an early trial in patients with IDDM, pramlintide given by continuous intravenous (IV) infusion caused significant delay of the gastric emptying rate during both the liquid and solid phases of a meal.[12]

In a double-blind, placebo-controlled, two-period crossover study, 18 male patients with IDDM were divided into two groups and assigned either an IV infusion of pramlintide (50 mcg/hour) or a placebo infusion for five hours.[9] Thirty minutes after injecting their morning dose of insulin subcutaneously, one group ingested a standardized meal of Sustacal, while the other group received a glucose load by IV infusion (300 mg/kg). A steady decline of plasma glucose levels in patients treated with pramlintide as compared to placebo-treated patients was demonstrated ($p = 0.0015$ versus placebo) for five hours following ingestion of an oral glucose load (Sustacal). In contrast, in patients receiving the

IV glucose load, a sharp postprandial rise in glucose occurred to almost the same extent in the pramlintide group as compared with placebo ($p = 0.54$). In this study, glycemic control was unaffected when glucose loads were administered IV, thus supporting the theory that pramlintide acts mainly by delaying gastric emptying and slowing the rate at which nutrients enter the circulation.

In a double-blind, placebo-controlled study in patients with IDDM, the effect of subcutaneous administration of pramlintide was assessed.[13] Patients were randomly assigned to receive injections of placebo, 30, 100, or 300 mcg pramlintide three times daily 30 minutes before meals for 14 days. All patients who received pramlintide, regardless of dose, exhibited a significant reduction in plasma glucose postprandially after 14 days of therapy. With the exception of the 300 mcg dose, peak plasma pramlintide concentrations were within or just slightly outside the physiological range for amylin.

Pramlintide has also been effective in reducing postprandial glucose levels in patients with NIDDM. In a randomized, double-blind, placebo-controlled crossover study, postprandial glucose elevations were significantly reduced for up to four hours following ingestion of a Sustacal meal in patients receiving pramlintide 100 mcg/hour by continuous IV infusion.[14] In addition, plasma insulin levels were also decreased in patients receiving pramlintide. This suggests that amylin is, at least in part, active in the regulation of the beta cell in patients with NIDDM.

The most common side effects of pramlintide are gastrointestinal in nature and are generally seen only with higher doses. In one study, 19 of 21 (90 percent) of patients receiving 300 mcg of pramlintide subcutaneously three times daily reported experiencing nausea with occasional episodes of emesis.[13] However, gastrointestinal symptoms were reported in 65 percent and 33 percent of patients receiving pramlintide 100 mcg and 30 mcg three times daily, respectively. Approximately 18 percent of patients in the placebo group reported experiencing gastrointestinal side effects.

Overall, pramlintide appears to be effective in reducing postprandial rises in glucose when administered by either IV infusion or subcutaneously. Adverse effects appear to occur less frequently at lower daily doses.[13] However, patient acceptance of and compliance with an agent that must be injected subcutaneously three times daily are also of concern. To avoid multiple daily injections, it will be imperative that pramlintide exhibit stability sufficient to allow mixing with insulin in the same syringe.

ENZYME INHIBITION

Voglibose and other Alpha-glucosidase inhibitors

Voglibose (AO-128; Takeda America) was isolated from *Streptomyces hygroscopius limoneus* and belongs to a class of drugs known as alpha-glucosidase inhibitors.[15] Currently, acarbose (Precose; Bayer) is the only agent in this category approved for use in the United States. The alpha-glucosidase enzyme is found in the brush border of the intestine and is necessary for the breakdown of di- and polysaccharides (e.g., sucrose, starch, dextrin) into monosaccharides. Therefore, inhibition of the alpha-glucosidase enzyme by voglibose results in a decreased absorption of complex carbohydrates and sugars.[16] In patients with diabetes, the delayed absorption of disaccharides leads to an attenuated rise in postprandial blood glucose concentration.

In addition to altering postprandial glucose concentrations, voglibose may also lower fasting blood glucose levels by yet another mechanism. Two intestinal peptide hormones known as gastric inhibitory polypeptide (GIP) and glucagon-like peptide (GLP) have been identified. These hormones are called *incretins*, which means they are mediators of insulin secretion from the endocrine pancreas in response to an oral nutrient intake.[17] Administration of an alpha-glucosidase inhibitor leads to a depression of GIP plasma levels, while increasing the plasma level of the insulintropic gut hormone GLP-1.[18]

The increase in release of GLP-1 after administration of voglibose along with a delayed increase in blood glucose postprandially may act together to improve overall glycemic control in patients with NIDDM. Indeed, the GLP-1 receptor in humans has been characterized and, theoretically, GLP-1 agonists for oral use could be designed. The practicality and limitations of this therapy have yet to be explored.[19]

The effects of voglibose on fasting blood glucose as well as its ability to stimulate secretion of GLP-1 were studied in a recent double-blind trial involving 72 healthy volunteers.[20] Six parallel groups of 12 volunteers received voglibose in oral doses of 0.5, 1.0, 2.0, or 5.0 mg, or placebo three times daily for seven days. Blood was drawn at preset intervals over 180 minutes on study Days -1, 1, and 7 to measure levels of glucose, insulin, C peptide, GIP, and GLP-1. Voglibose was associated with a dose-dependent, significant reduction in postprandial increases of insulin, glucose, and C peptide when compared to placebo. The 0.5 mg and 1.0 mg doses had a more pronounced effect on blood glucose and insulin concentrations on Day 7 as compared to Day 1. The glucose-lowering effect of the 2.0 mg and 5.0 mg doses was already maximal on Day 1. Volunteers treated with voglibose 5 mg three times daily experienced reduced postprandial insulin concentrations up to 60 to 70 percent of maximum concentrations before voglibose treatment.

With respect to GIP concentrations, all doses of voglibose showed a decrease that was significant from placebo for both Day 1 and Day 7. In contrast, GLP-1 secretion was enhanced to greater than 80 percent above control levels ($p < 0.001$) after the first voglibose dose of 1.0 mg. On Day 7, GLP-1 concentrations were shown to be greater than 90 percent above controls. No further increase was noted with the 2 and 5 mg doses.

Voglibose is approved in Japan for treating patients with NIDDM; clinical studies in the United States for patients with NIDDM are ongoing.[15] Like acarbose, voglibose is poorly absorbed from the intestinal tract, which increases the incidence of gastrointestinal side effects. In the aforementioned study, 59.7 percent of voglibose-treated patients (versus 5.6 percent on placebo) reported occurrence of gastrointestinal events, such as stool loss, diarrhea, meteorism (distention by gas in the abdomen or intestines), and upset stomach.[20] These types of side effects occur due to the malabsorptive syndrome that is set up when carbohydrates are not absorbed from the upper intestine, which leads to a greater amount of carbohydrates present in the lower intestine.[21] These same symptoms are often noted in general in patients with NIDDM. In both clinical Phase I and II studies of patients with NIDDM, the most commonly observed side effects were meteorism and diarrhea.[21] However, these side effects seem to occur early in therapy and lessen with time. This may confirm the need for these types of drugs to be started at low, infrequent doses and gradually titrated upward. Also, patients should be advised to avoid diets high in simple sugars and to increase their intake of starches and high-fiber foods.

Other drugs in this category in various stages of development include miglitol (Baym1099; Bayer), which is a second-generation alpha-glucosidase inhibitor derived from 1-desoxynojirimycin.[22] Miglitol is a potent, competitive inhibitor of sucrase and glucoamylase. However, unlike acarbose, desoxynojirimycin compounds undergo almost complete absorption from the small intestine.[23] Although it was thought that this might decrease the severity and frequency of gastrointestinal side effects, a small study ($n = 36$) of patients with NIDDM failed to support this theory.[23] In other clinical studies of both patients with IDDM and NIDDM, miglitol demonstrated a significant decrease in postprandial blood glucose at a dose of 50 to 100 mg three times daily.[24] Higher doses were associated with an increased incidence of flatulence, abdominal distention, and diarrhea.

Emiglitate is yet another desoxynojirimycin derivative (Bayer).[25] It is more potent and longer acting than either acarbose or miglitol. However, superior control of postprandial hyperglycemia in comparison to the previous agents has not been demonstrated, and the gastrointestinal

side effects have occurred with greater frequency. Therefore, this drug is no longer in development. Other compounds have also been synthesized compounds that appear, at least in early studies, to have potent alpha-glucosidase inhibitory activity.[26]

AGENTS THAT INCREASE INSULIN SENSITIVITY

Resistance to the effects of insulin is a common feature among patients with NIDDM.[3,27] Chronic hyperglycemia leads to increased secretion of insulin from the beta-cells of the pancreas. This increased secretion of insulin by the beta-cells over a long period of time leads to beta-cell exhaustion and resulting hyperglycemia.[3] Agents that not only decrease plasma glucose but also decrease insulin levels should aid in increasing insulin sensitivity.

Insulin-like Growth Factors

Insulin-like growth factors (IGFs) are polypeptide compounds that are structurally related to proinsulin. They were formally referred to as *somatomedin-C*.[28] Endogenous growth factors are found in varying concentrations in most all body tissues and circulate via binding proteins (IGFBPs). To date, six IGFBPs have been identified. However, only three—IGFBP-I, -II, and -III—have been well characterized in humans.[29-31]

IGF-I is a 70 amino acid peptide that mimics the effects of insulin on carbohydrate metabolism and glucose concentration. Using recombinant deoxyribonucleic acid (DNA) technology, human IGF-I (rhIGF-I; Genentech) has been synthesized and is being studied for the treatment of IDDM and NIDDM and other diseases.[32] In vitro studies demonstrate that IGF-I enhances glucose uptake, stimulates protein and lipid synthesis, and inhibits lipolysis.[33-35] These effects are mediated through the interaction of IGF-I with the tissue IGF-I receptor. IGF-I may also exhibit crossover stimulation with the insulin receptor. On a molar basis, IGF-I is only 6 percent as potent with respect to glucose-lowering effects as insulin.[36] However, studies in animals have demonstrated that rhIGF-I has effects similar to insulin in its ability to stimulate glucose uptake, glycogen synthesis, and glycolysis. Glucose uptake was restored to near normal in two insulin-dependent animal models when given an infusion of IGF-I.[37] In contrast, glucose uptake did not normalize in the same animals when given an infusion of insulin. However, in hyperinsulinemic, insulin-resistant animals, rhIGF-I appeared less effective with respect to glucose metabolism stimulation.[38]

In humans, rhIGF-I appears effective in treating both patients with IDDM and those with NIDDM. IGF-I may be administered by IV infusion or subcutaneously. The half-life of IGF-I is about 16 to 23 hours with a first-order pharmacokinetic profile. IGF-I is highly bound to IGFBP, with a relatively low volume of distribution of 0.2 to 0.36 l/kg.[39]

In a double-blind, placebo-controlled study, either rhIGF-I (40 mcg/kg) or a saline solution was administered subcutaneously to adolescent subjects with IDDM.[40] Subjects were also given insulin by infusion in a dose sufficient to achieve euglycemia. Exogenous administration of rhIGF-I resulted in a decrease in the amount of insulin required to maintain euglycemia by 7 to 38 percent; plasma-free insulin concentrations were also decreased by 50 percent. Another similar study found that insulin requirements in IDDM patients receiving an rhIGF-I infusion were decreased by 60 percent.[41] These data appear to support the theory that the action of IGF-I is due at least in part to enhancing insulin sensitivity.

One characteristic common to most patients with NIDDM is hyperinsulinemia as well as hyperglycemia. This hyperinsulinemia is thought to contribute to the development of atherosclerosis as well as other microvascular complications, including retinopathy.[2] Patients with NIDDM who have failed to achieve glycemic control with diet, exercise, and oral medications must be treated with exogenous insulin. This insulin, usually in supraphysiologic doses, further compounds the problems associated with hyperinsulinemia. It is thought that administration of IGF-I to patients

with NIDDM will not only serve to help lower blood glucose levels but will also decrease insulin levels and, thus, help slow or halt the progression of diabetic complications.[29]

In one study, Zenobi et al. studied eight patients with NIDDM who were previously treated with either diet alone or diet and an oral agent.[42] Patients were given rhIGF-I at 120 mcg/kg body weight subcutaneously twice daily for five days. All subjects were evaluated for five control days before drug administration on Day 6. The administration of rhIGF-I caused a significant decrease in mean fasting glucose and insulin concentrations. Area under the curve was also significantly decreased for postprandial glucose and insulin levels.

In a study by Schalch et al., 12 patients with NIDDM received subcutaneous injections of rhIGF-I in doses ranging from 90 to 160 mcg/kg twice daily for five days.[43] As in the previously cited study, there was a significant decrease in area under the curve for both plasma glucose concentration and postprandial glucose (decreased by 30 to 35 percent of controls). Plasma insulin concentrations were also decreased by 40 to 50 percent.

At the time of this writing, rhIGF-I is still being evaluated in large, controlled clinical studies. Of concern are the possible untoward side effects that may accompany long-term rhIGF-I administration, specifically, the development or progression of microvascular complications, such as retinopathy. Because it is a growth factor, rhIGF-I has the potential to stimulate smooth muscle cell proliferation.[44] It also has vasodilatory properties, which may increase capillary leakage in response to increased blood flow and further contribute to the development of proliferative diabetic retinopathy (PDR) and nephropathy. IGF-I levels of over 900 diabetic patients who were diagnosed at the age of 30 or older were measured in a study by Dills et al.[45] When controlling for other factors, such as duration of diabetes and glycosylated hemoglobin, higher levels of IGF-I were found to be associated with an increased frequency of PDR ($p = 0.025$) in insulin users. In patients not using insulin, PDR and moderate non-PDR were also associated with increased levels of IGF-I ($p = 0.08$). However, many other studies have failed to show a correlation between IGF-I levels and retinopathy.[46,47] A six-year study evaluating the association of IGF-I to the incidence and progression of retinopathy in 2,990 diabetic patients of varying ages failed to find such an association.[48] However, retinopathy and other microvascular complications (nephropathy and neuropathy) should continue to be evaluated in patients, especially with long-term use of IGF-I.

Other side effects that have been noted are those related to muscle and joint pain. A small study ($n = 7$) conducted by Jabri et al. was discontinued early because patients developed frequent recurrences of arthralgias, myalgias, flushing, and dyspnea.[49] However, patients in this study were given doses of 120 to 160 mcg/kg twice daily, which are among the highest in the literature. It is important to realize that rhIGF-I should always be dosed based on lean muscle mass and not total body weight.

Thiazolidinediones

Thiazolidinediones represent a new class of agents for the treatment of NIDDM. This group of drugs has in common a 2,4-dione nuclear structure.[50] Altering the side chains has produced agents, including troglitazone (CS-045), for which FDA approval is expected soon, pioglitazone, and ciglitazone, that lower glucose as well as insulin and triglyceride levels.[51] The mechanism of action for this class is not completely understood but is thought to be due to a receptor and postreceptor effect on peripheral tissue (e.g., fat, muscle, and liver) responses to insulin.[52,53] Animal studies with both troglitazone and ciglitazone have demonstrated that the compounds decrease plasma levels of glucose, while lowering insulin levels as well, in a dose-dependent manner.[54] The thiazolidinediones do not enhance insulin secretion and have no effect on glycemic control in insulinopenic animals, making them ineffective in the treatment of IDDM.

One study evaluated the effects of troglitazone on glucose concentrations and insulin levels in response to an oral glucose load.[55] Nineteen patients with NIDDM whose glycemic control was noted as unsatisfactory on either diet alone or diet plus oral agents were studied. After an eight-week observation period, patients were then started on oral doses of troglitazone at 200 mg twice daily for 12 weeks. Patients were allowed to continue their previous treatment (i.e., diet alone +/- oral agents) with the troglitazone added to this therapy. Eight patients were treated with troglitazone alone, and 11 were treated with troglitazone plus a sulfonylurea. A glucose tolerance test was administered both before and after therapy with troglitazone. Fasting plasma glucose was significantly decreased after troglitazone therapy ($p < 0.001$), as was the hemoglobin HbA$_{1C}$ ($p < 0.005$). Fasting insulin levels also decreased after treatment with troglitazone ($p < 0.05$). Given that glycemic control was favorably affected while insulin levels were decreased, these data confirm the earlier conclusion that the mechanism of action of this compound includes increasing insulin sensitivity. Similar results were reported by Suter et al., except that 3 out of 11 patients did not show a statistically significant response in reduction of hyperglycemia.[51] These three patients also had the lowest insulin-secretory profiles of all the patients. Presumably, since troglitazone exerts its effects via increasing insulin sensitivity, patients must have adequate circulating levels of insulin for drugs of this class to be effective in decreasing hyperglycemia. However, this hypothesis needs to be studied further in a larger number of patients.

If it is found that thiazolidinediones have no significant effect on glycemic control for patients with low levels of circulating insulin, their place in therapy will then be more clearly defined. Patients in this category might receive more benefit from an insulin secretagogue, such as a sulfonylurea. However, in patients with adequate insulin stores, thiazolidinediones may be beneficial when used alone. These compounds may also eventually be used in combination with an oral sulfonylurea or insulin for patients who manifest signs of both decreased insulin secretion and decreased insulin sensitivity.

•   •   •

Many new compounds for the treatment of IDDM and NIDDM are currently being evaluated in clinical trials. A majority of these new agents belongs to entirely new classes of agents not previously marketed. New therapies that act by different mechanisms of action than what is currently available may add favorably to the present armamentarium of agents available. It may soon be possible to "tailor-make" antidiabetic therapy depending on the predominant impairments, whether this be lack of insulin secretion or a decreased insulin sensitivity.

REFERENCES

1. The Diabetes Control and Complications Trial Research Group, "The Effect of Intensive Treatment of Diabetes on the Development and Progression of Long-term Complications in Insulin-dependent Diabetes Mellitus," *New England Journal of Medicine* 329 (1993): 977–986.

2. American Diabetes Association, "Implications of the Diabetes Control and Complications Trial," *Diabetes* 42 (1993): 1,555–1,558.

3. R.A. Defronzo, "The Triumvirate: beta-cell, Muscle, Liver. A Collusion Responsible for NIDDM," *Diabetes* 37 (1988): 667–687.

4. S.P. Clissold, and C. Edwards, "Acarbose: A Preliminary Review of Its Pharmacodynamic and Pharmacokinetic Properties, and Therapeutic Potential," *Drugs* 35 (1988): 214–243.

5. G.S. Cooper et al., "Purification and Characterization of a Peptide from Amyloid-rich Pancreas of Type 2 Diabetic Patients," *Proceedings of the National Academy of Science USA* 84 (1987): 8,628–8,632.

6. B.R. Gedulin et al., "Dose-response for Glucagonostatic Effect of Amylin in Rats," unpublished manuscript.

7. J. Wahren et al., "Effect of Protein Ingestion on Splanchnic and Leg Metabolism in Normal Man and in Diabetes," *Journal of Clinical Investigations* 56 (1975): 1,250.

8. J.G. Schwartz et al., "Rapid Gastric Emptying of a Solid Pancake Meal in Type 2 Diabetic Patients," *Diabetes Care* 19 (1996): 468–471.

9. O.G. Kolterman et al., "Reduction of Postprandial Hyperglycemia in Subjects with IDDM by Intravenous Infusion of AC137, a Human Amylin Analogue," *Diabetes Care* 18, no. 8 (1995): 1,179–1,182.

10. A. Clark et al., "Islet Amyloid Formed from Diabetes-associated Peptide May Be Pathogenic in Type-2 Diabetes," *Lancet* ii (1987): 231–234.

11. A.A. Young et al., "Gastric Emptying Is Accelerated in Diabetic BB Rats and Is Slowed by Subcutaneous Injections of Amylin," *Diabetologia* 38 (1995): 642–648.

12. I. Macdonald et al., "Infusion of the Human Amylin Analogue, AC137, Delays Gastric Emptying in Men with IDDM," *Diabetologia* 38, suppl. 1 (1995): A32. Abstract.

13. O.G. Kolterman et al., "Effect of 14 Days' Subcutaneous Administration of the Human Amylin Analogue, Pramlintide (AC137), on an Intravenous Insulin Challenge and Response to a Standard Liquid Meal in Patients with IDDM," *Diabetologia* 39 (1996): 492–499.

14. O.G. Kolterman et al., "The Effect of Pramlintide (AC137) on Postprandial Hyperglycemia in Patients with Type II Diabetes," *Diabetologia* 38, suppl. 1 (1995): A193. Abstract.

15. H. Odaka, and T. Matsuo, "Effect of a Disaccharidase Inhibitor, AO-128, on Post-prandial Hyperglycemia in Rats," *Journal of Japan Society of Nutrition, Food and Science* 45 (1992): 27–31.

16. S. Horii et al., "Synthesis and Alpha-D-glucosidase Inhibitory Activity of N-Substituted Valiolamine Derivatives as Potential Oral Antidiabetic Agents," *Journal of Medicinal Chemistry* 29 (1986): 1,038–1,046.

17. J.C. Brown, "Enteroinsular Axis." in *Gut Peptides*, eds. U.H. Walsh and G.J. Dockray (New York: Raven Press, 1994), 765–803.

18. R. Ebert, and W. Creutzfeldt, "Decreased GIP Secretion through Impairment of Absorption," *Frontiers of Hormonal Research* 7 (1980): 192–201.

19. B. Thorens et al., "Cloning and Functional Expression of the Human Islet GLP-1 Receptor: Demonstration that Extendin-4 is an Agonist and Extendin-9 (9-39) an Antagonist of the Receptor," *Diabetes* 42 (1993): 1,678–1,682.

20. B. Goke et al., "Voglibose (AO-128) Is an Efficient α-Glucosidase Inhibitor and Mobilizes the Endogenous GLP-1 Reserve," *Digestion* 56 (1995): 493–501.

21. S. Baba, "Diabetes: Focus on alpha-Glucosidase Inhibitors," in *International Trends in Drug Treatment* (Tokyo: Churchill Livingstone, 1994).

22. R.R. Holman et al., "Post-Prandial Glycaemic Reduction by an α-glucosidase Inhibitor in Type 2 Diabetic

Patients with Therapeutically Attained Basal Normo-glycaemia," *Diabetes Research* 18 (1991): 149–153.

23. P.J. Kingma et al., "α-Glucosidase Inhibition by Miglitol in NIDDM Patients," *Diabetes Care* 15 (1992): 478–483.

24. N. Katsilambros et al., "A Double-Blind Study on the Efficacy and Tolerance of a New Alpha-glucosidase Inhibitor in Type 2 Diabetics," *Arzneim Forsch* 36 (1986): 1,136–1,138.

25. R. Bressler, and D. Johnson, "New Pharmacological Approaches to Therapy of NIDDM," *Diabetes Care* 15, no. 6 (1992): 792–805.

26. B.L. Rhinehart et al., "Inhibition of Intestinal Disaccharidases and Suppression of Blood Glucose by a New α-Glucohydrolase Inhibitor-MDL 25,637," *Journal of Pharmacology and Therapeutics* 241 (1987): 915–920.

27. H. Yki-Jarvinen, "Acute and Chronic Effects of Hyperglycaemia on Glucose Metabolism," *Diabetologia* 33 (1990): 579–585.

28. M.E. Svoboda et al., "Purification of Somatomedin-C from Human Plasma: Chemical and Biological Properties, Partial Sequence Analysis, and Relationship to Other Somatomedins," *Biochemistry* 19 (1980): 790–797.

29. M.N. Rechler, and S.P. Nissley, "Insulin-like Growth Factors," In *Peptide Growth Factors and Their Receptors*, 1st ed, eds. M.B. Sporn and A.B. Roberts (New York: Springer-Verlag, 1990), 263–367.

30. M.S. Lewitt, "Role of the Insulin-like Growth Factors in the Endocrine Control of Glucose Homeostasis," *Diabetes Research and Clinical Practice* 23 (1994): 3–15.

31. G. Lamson et al., "IGF Binding Proteins: Structural and Molecular Relationships," *Growth Factors* 5 (1991): 19–28.

32. K. Cusi, and R.A. DeFronzo, "Treatment of NIDDM, IDDM, and Other Insulin-resistant States with IGF-I," *Diabetes Reviews* 3, no. 2 (1995): 206–236.

33. E.R. Froesch, and J. Zapf, "Insulin-like Growth Factors and Insulin: Comparative Aspects," *Diabetologia* 28 (1985): 485–493.

34. W. Kiess et al., "Growth Hormone and Insulin-like Growth Factor I: Basic Aspects," in *Growth Hormone and Insulin-Like Growth Factor I in Human and Experimental Diabetes*, eds A. Flyvbjerg et al. (New York: Wiley, 1993), 22.

35. R.C. Baxter, and J.L. Martin, "Binding Proteins for the Insulin-like Growth Factors: Structure, Regulation and Function," *Progressive Growth Factor Research* 1 (1989): 49–68.

36. H.P. Guler et al., "Short-term Metabolic Effects of Recombinant Human Insulin-like Growth Factor I in Healthy Adults," *New England Journal of Medicine* 317 (1987):137–140.

37. L. Rossetti et al., "Metabolic Effects of IGF-I in Diabetic Rats," *Diabetes* 40 (1991): 444–448.

38. M.A. Cascieri et al., "Impaired Insulin Growth Factor I: Mediated Stimulation of Glucose Incorporation into Glycogen in Vivo in the Ob/ob Mouse," *Diabetologia* 32 (1989): 342–347.

39. A. Grahnen et al., "Pharmacokinetics of Recombinant Human Insulin-like Growth Factor I Given Subcutaneously to Healthy Volunteers and to Patients with Growth Hormone Receptor Deficiency," *Academy of Pediatrics* Supplement 391, (1993): 9–13.

40. T.D. Cheetham et al., "The Effects of Recombinant Human Insulin-like Growth Factor I Administration on Growth Hormone Levels and Insulin Requirements in Adolescents with Insulin Dependent Diabetes Mellitus," *Diabetologia* 36, (1993): 678–681.

41. M.A. Bach et al., "The Effects of Subcutaneous Insulin-like Growth Factor-I infusion in Insulin-dependent Diabetes Mellitus," *Journal of Clinical Endocrinology and Metabolism* 79, (1994): 1,040–1,045.

42. P.D. Zenobi et al., "Insulin-like Growth Factor-I Improves Glucose and Lipid Metabolism in Type 2 Diabetes Mellitus," *Journal of Clinical Investigation* 90 (1992): 2,234–2,241.

43. D.S. Schalch et al., "Short-term Effects of Recombinant Human Insulin-like Growth Factor I on Metabolic Control in Patients with Type II Diabetes Mellitus," *Journal of Clinical Endocrinology and Metabolism* 77 (1993): 1,563–1,568.

44. K.E. Bornfeldt, and H.J. Arnqvist, "Actions of Insulin-like Growth Factor-I and Insulin in Vascular Smooth Muscle: Receptor Interaction and Growth-Promoting. In *Growth Hormone and Insulin-Like Growth Factor I in Human and Experimental Diabetes*, eds. A. Glyvbjerg et al. (New York: Wiley, 1993), 159–192.

45. D.G. Dills et al., "Association of Elevated IGF-I Levels with Increased Retinopathy in Late-onset Diabetes," *Diabetes* 40 (1991): 1,725–1,730.

46. H. Jarvelainen et al., "Insulin-like Growth Factor-I in Type 2 (Non–insulin-dependent) Diabetics with Myocardial Infarction and Without Macroangiopathy," *Atherosclerosis* 59 (1986): 335–340.

47. Q. Wang et al., "Is Insulin-like Growth Factor Predictive of 6-Year Incidence and Progression of Diabetic Retinopathy?" *Diabetes* 43 suppl.1 (1994): 25A.

48. Q. Wang et al., "Does Insulin-like Growth Factor I Predict Incidence and Progression of Diabetic Retinopathy?" *Diabetes* 44 (1995): 161–164.

49. N. Jabri et al., "Adverse Effects of Recombinant Human Insulin-like Growth Factor I in Obese Insulin-resistant Type II Diabetic Patients," *Diabetes* 43 (1994): 369–374.

50. D.J. Eckland, "Thiazolidinediones: A New Class of Antidiabetic Agent," in *Proceedings of International Conference on Diabetes: Current Perspectives* (London: New Medicines, 1994).

51. S.L. Suter et al., "Metabolic Effects of New Oral Hypoglycemic Agent CS-045 in Subjects," *Diabetes Care* 15 (1992): 193–203.

52. T. Fujiwara et al., "Characterization of a New Oral Antidiabetic Agent CS-045: Studies in KK and Ob/ob Mice and Zuker Fatty Rats," *Diabetes* 37 (1988): 1,549–1,558.

53. T.P. Ciaraldi et al., "In Vitro Studies on the Action of CS-045: A New Antidiabetic Agent," *Metabolism* 39 (1990): 1,056–1,062.

54. T. Fujita et al., "Reduction of Insulin-resistance in Obese and/or Diabetic Animals by 5-[4-(1-methylcyclohexylmethoxy)-benzyl] thiazolidine-2,4-dione (ADD-3878, U-63287, Ciglitazone), a New Antidiabetic Agent," *Diabetes* 32 (1983): 804–810.

55. Y. Iwamota et al., "Effect of New Oral Antidiabetic Agent CS-045 on Glucose Tolerance and Insulin Secretion in Patients with NIDDM," *Diabetes Care* 14, no. 11 (1991): 1,083–1,086.

Managing Therapy and Adverse Effects with Antihyperglycemic Agents: A Focus on Metformin and Acarbose

Beth Bryles Phillips, PharmD

Metformin and acarbose are novel antihyperglycemic agents indicated for the treatment of non–insulin-dependent diabetes mellitus. These agents offer new therapeutic options to control hyperglycemia that were previously unavailable. Common to both agents is a relatively high incidence of gastrointestinal adverse effects. Initiating therapy at a low dose and slowly titrating to therapeutic response may be the most effective way to minimize associated adverse effects. Recognition and proper management of these possible adverse effects can optimize therapy and maximize the potential for successful outcomes with these agents while limiting drug noncompliance. Key words: *acarbose, adverse effects, compliance, diabetes mellitus, metformin*

The compliance rate for drug therapy used to treat chronic disease states, such as diabetes mellitus, is estimated to be only 50 percent.[1] Not only does noncompliance result in failure to reach therapeutic outcomes, but it is also costly to the health care system. It is estimated that the total cost of pharmacologic noncompliance is more than 33 billion dollars.[2] Perhaps of most importance and a key determinant of noncompliance is adverse drug reactions.[3] These issues may be particularly important with regard to two relatively new agents available for the treatment of non–insulin-dependent diabetes mellitus (NIDDM), metformin (Glucophage, Bristol-Myers Squibb Company) and acarbose (Precose, Bayer Corporation). Metformin and acarbose are associated with a considerable number of adverse effects, which are most notably gastrointestinal in nature.[4] Of note, these adverse effects may have led to abnormally high dropout rates in clinical trials designed to evaluate these agents in patients with NIDDM.[5–7] Due to the much-needed benefits these agents confer to

many patients with NIDDM, a concerted effort should be made to control or minimize the incidence of unwanted side effects.

NOVEL ANTIHYPERGLYCEMIC AGENTS

Until recently, pharmacologic therapy for the estimated 12 million Americans with NIDDM centered around oral sulfonylureas with progression to insulin once oral sulfonylureas alone failed to control blood glucose concentrations.[8] Metformin and acarbose offer new therapeutic options that were previously unavailable. In contrast to insulin and oral sulfonylureas, both of these agents lower blood glucose concentrations without raising systemic insulin levels and consequently are not expected to cause hypoglycemic reactions or weight gain.[9,10]

Metformin is a biguanide antihyperglycemic agent structurally similar to phenformin. Phenformin was used several years ago until the unacceptable high risk of lactic acidosis was realized.[11] Metformin decreases both fasting and postprandial blood glucose concentrations. It lowers fasting blood glucose primarily by reducing hepatic glucose output.[12] In addition, metformin decreases intestinal absorption of glucose and improves glucose uptake and utilization in peripheral tissues.[13] These actions are largely responsible for the ability of metformin to lower fasting plasma glucose concentrations and glycosylated hemoglobin as seen in recent clinical trials.[7,14]

Acarbose is part of an exciting new class of agents used in the treatment of NIDDM, the alpha-glucosidase inhibitors. It is currently the only alpha-glucosidase inhibitor available in the United States and has a unique mechanism of action. Not only does acarbose inhibit alpha-glucosidase enzymes, but it also inhibits pancreatic alpha-amylase, which ultimately leads to a delay in the absorption of glucose from the gut.[15] Acarbose is comparable in structure to oligosaccharides, which are normal products of systemic starch degradation.[16] Pancreatic alpha-amylase is responsible for the degradation of starches into oligosaccharides.[15] Alpha-glucosidase enzymes, which include glucoamylase, sucrase, maltase, and isomaltase, normally metabolize complex sugars, such as oligosaccharides and disaccharides, into simple sugars, such as glucose and fructose.[10] Although alpha-glucosidase enzymes are present throughout the lower gastrointestinal tract, the greatest concentration of these enzymes is located in the brush border of the small intestine. Acarbose competitively and reversibly binds to and inhibits only those enzymes located in the brush border. As a result, complex carbohydrates normally broken down in the brush border are passed down into the distal ileum and later into the large intestine where they are digested, in part, by alpha-glucosidase enzymes and colonic bacteria, respectively.[16] By prolonging the digestion of complex carbohydrates and reducing the rate of glucose absorption, acarbose blunts the postprandial peak in blood glucose concentrations. Consequently, acarbose reduces glycosylated hemoglobin concentrations

and may also produce modest reductions in fasting blood glucose levels.[6,17] Postprandial plasma glucose concentrations are effectively reduced by acarbose as carbohydrate consumption comprises approximately one half of the normal Western diet, and approximately 90 percent of these carbohydrates are derived from starch and sucrose.[10]

MANAGEMENT OF ADVERSE EFFECTS

One of the most important sequelae of adverse effects is the impact on compliance. This is especially important with regard to the treatment of diabetes mellitus, as control of hyperglycemia has been shown to postpone and reduce the development of nephropathy, neuropathy, and retinopathy in insulin-dependent diabetes mellitus (IDDM).[18] Although not proven for NIDDM, it has been suggested that control of hyperglycemia will produce comparable results on microvascular complications.[19] Education, early recognition, and management of potential adverse effects will maximize the chance for successful outcomes with respect to therapy.

Although metformin and acarbose are devoid of many of the unwanted systemic adverse effects associated with insulin and oral sulfonylureas, most notably hypoglycemia and hyperinsulinemia, each of these agents is associated with its own unique adverse effect profile. Withdrawal rates due to adverse effects have been reported to be up to 11 percent for metformin[7,20] and up to 19 percent for acarbose in clinical trials.[5,21] Drug-induced gastrointestinal symptoms were the most frequently reported adverse effects from both agents by the patients studied.[5–7,15,20,22] Gastrointestinal adverse effects were also the most common reason for early discontinuation of therapy and patient withdrawal from clinical trials.[5–7] Although the outcomes of the clinical trials do not always mirror clinical practice, these points highlight the need for proper recognition and management of potential adverse effects that may lead to drug noncompliance in the clinical setting.

METFORMIN

Gastrointestinal Adverse Effects

Gastrointestinal adverse effects are the most frequently reported adverse events associated with the use of metformin, occurring in up to 30 percent of patients. Symptoms commonly reported include diarrhea, nausea, vomiting, abdominal bloating, flatulence, and anorexia.[22] Of these, diarrhea was the most frequent gastrointestinal symptom reported.[4,7] In a recent evaluation of 289 obese patients who received metformin at a dose of 850 mg three times daily or placebo, 8 percent had complaints of severe diarrhea, and 4 percent had complaints of severe nausea.[7] There is some evidence to suggest the diarrhea associated with metformin therapy may not be dose-related. This finding was reported in a British study that evaluated 285 patients by questionnaire in a diabetes clinic. Diarrhea was noted in 20 percent of patients receiving metformin therapy, and there was no difference in incidence of diarrhea at different daily dosages.[23]

The key to the management of gastrointestinal side effects associated with metformin is to start with low doses and titrate slowly.[4,13] It has been suggested that doses as low as 500 mg daily may be an appropriate starting dose for some patients.[4] Titration of doses should not occur at a rate faster than one tablet per week.[22] These effects may also be minimized by administering metformin with food. If gastrointestinal effects (e.g., diarrhea) persist, a reduction in dose or even discontinuation of therapy may be warranted to provide relief of symptoms.[4]

Recent evidence from a European trial suggests gastrointestinal adverse effects and metallic taste may subside over time. This multicenter trial evaluated 1,823 patients with NIDDM whose blood glucose was not adequately controlled with diet and a sulfonylurea. Patients received metformin in doses of 850 to 2,550 mg daily for 12 weeks. At the end of the 12-week trial, less than 1 percent of patients had gastrointestinal complaints compared to 7 percent of patients at the initiation of therapy. Similarly, no patients had complaints of metallic taste at the end of the 12 weeks compared to 16 patients at the onset of therapy. Overall, 14.2 percent of patients experienced gastrointestinal adverse effects. However, data on gastrointestinal effects were only available on 7 percent of patients. These findings suggest that tolerance may develop to these adverse effects over time.[24] Therefore, a management option in those patients who have mild to moderate adverse effects is to continue therapy in an attempt to develop tolerance.

Lactic Acidosis

Perhaps the most feared and potentially severe complication of metformin therapy is lactic acidosis. Fortunately, the frequency of this event is relatively rare, with a reported incidence of 0 to 0.08 cases/1,000 patient years.[13] However, the mortality rate in patients who develop lactic acidosis may be as high as 50 percent.[4] The mortality risk is reported to be 0 to 0.024/1,000 patient years.[13] Lactic acidosis is a metabolic acidosis characterized by a high anion gap (greater than 15 mmol/l), pH less than 7.25, and a plasma lactate concentration greater than 5 mmol/l.[4] Symptoms are nonspecific and may be difficult to distinguish as clinically significant. The most common symptom is vomiting, followed by somnolence, nausea, epigastric pain, anorexia, hyperpnea, lethargy, diarrhea, thirst, muscle weakness, and cramping.[25]

Phenformin is associated with an estimated risk of lactic acidosis 10 to 15 times higher than that of metformin.[4,13,26] It is thought that differences in metabolism and mechanisms of action account for the difference in risk between these two agents.[4,7,12,13,27] In contrast to phenformin, it is uncertain whether metformin induces lactic acidosis under normal circumstances.[4,7,13,26] Instead, it may indirectly enhance the development of lactic acidosis when other conditions exist that can cause accumulation of metformin (e.g., renal dysfunction), decrease lactate clearance (e.g., hepatic disease), or increase lactate production (e.g., conditions associated with reduced tissue perfusion).[4,26] It is thought that metformin may promote lactic acidosis through the inhibition of hepatic gluconeogenesis, which prevents the conversion of lactate to glucose.[25] In contrast, phenformin may prevent peripheral glucose oxidation and stimulate peripheral lactate production, which contributes to the development of lactic acidosis.[7] There is evidence to suggest that metformin does not raise fasting plasma lactate concentrations and does not stimulate the release of lactate from muscle.[12]

A Swedish study designed to evaluate the risk of lactic acidosis between 1977 and 1991 with metformin was conducted. This investigation revealed over the study period a cumulative index of 0.6 cases of associated acidosis per 10,000 patient years.[26] Almost all of the patients included in this retrospective study had serious concomitant cardiovascular diseases and were diagnosed with several other diseases. Only 1 patient of the 18 did not have renal insufficiency at the time of diagnosis. The mean age of these patients was 72 ± 7 years. In five patients, the onset of lactic acidosis was quick and occurred in less than 30 days after initiation of treatment. In others, therapy was ongoing for more than two years before the onset of acidosis.

Every effort possible should be made to prevent the development of lactic acidosis in patients receiving metformin. In most reported cases of lactic acidosis, a contraindication to metformin therapy was present. The most common contraindication noted was renal insufficiency, defined as a serum creatinine greater than 1.4 mg/dL in females or greater than 1.5 mg/dL in males.[22,26,28] In addition, it is important to realize that any major illness causing reduced tissue perfusion or hypoxia (e.g., hypotension) can also predispose patients to the development of lactic acidosis by promoting the formation of lactate.[28] Other contraindications to metformin therapy include severe hepatic disease, respiratory insufficiency, severe coronary artery disease (e.g., acute myocardial infarction), alcoholism, history of lactic acidosis, use of intravenous radiographic contrast agents, and pregnancy.[4,9,28] It is recommended that metformin therapy be avoided in chronic disease states associated with an increased risk of lactic acidosis

(e.g., renal insufficiency or severe hepatic disease) or temporarily discontinued in cases of acute illness (e.g., acute myocardial infarction or sepsis).[4,9] The management of lactic acidosis is controversial and not clearly defined in the medical literature. In general, management revolves around correction of the acidosis and hemodialysis in an attempt to remove excess metformin, lactate, and ketones from the systemic circulation.[4,25] Most importantly, patients should be educated on the signs and symptoms of this disorder.

Impaired Vitamin B12 and Folate Absorption

Reduced vitamin B12 concentrations were reported in 7 percent of patients receiving metformin in one trial, although none of these patients was symptomatic. In addition, only a few cases of megaloblastic anemia associated with metformin therapy have been reported. Patients with insufficient intake or absorption of vitamin B12 or calcium may be predisposed to developing these lowered concentrations, which are thought to be caused by an impaired absorption.[22] Although there was some initial concern of impaired folate absorption, a more recent trial found no significant decreases in serum folate concentrations.[3,22] Periodic monitoring for signs and symptoms of megaloblastic anemia and reduced vitamin B12 concentrations is warranted. If reduced concentrations develop, management consists of supplementation or discontinuation of therapy, if needed.[22,28]

Metallic Taste

Alterations in taste have been associated with the use of metformin.[20,22] In one study, metallic taste was reported in 11 percent of 144 patients.[21] It has been suggested that the alteration in taste may be due to the accumulation of metformin in the saliva.[22]

Hypoglycemia

Unlike the oral sulfonylureas, metformin does not stimulate the release of insulin and is not expected to cause hypoglycemia. This expectation is based on its unique mechanism of action. However, hypoglycemic reactions have occurred when metformin was administered concomitantly with oral sulfonylureas or insulin.[22]

ACARBOSE

With the exception of drug-related effects on the gastrointestinal system, acarbose has been noted to cause very few systemic adverse effects. Early clinical trials evaluating acarbose therapy for up to five years found no clinically significant variations in hematologic or biochemical functions.[10] However, headache and alterations in some laboratory parameters, including liver function tests, have been reported.[21,29] Minimal absorption of orally administered acarbose may account for this finding.[29] Approximately 1 percent of each dose of acarbose is systemically absorbed, and approximately 35 percent of each dose is metabolized in the intestine by bacteria and digestive enzymes.[15,29] A summary of reported adverse effects in recent controlled clinical trials evaluating acarbose therapy for up to one year in patients with NIDDM are located in Table 1.

Although the drop-out rates have been reported to be up to 19 percent for patients receiving acarbose therapy in recent clinical trials,[5,6,17,21,30] there is some evidence to suggest that acarbose has greater tolerability in general practice.[31] A Canadian postmarketing surveillance study of 10,462 patients with IDDM or NIDDM recently reported that only 2.9 percent of patients stopped therapy due to acarbose-induced adverse effects over a 12-week period. A majority of patients (78.6 percent) reported no adverse effects during the evaluation period using doses between 150 to 300 mg daily. The authors attributed this lower than expected incidence of adverse effects and greater tolerability of acarbose therapy to the fact that the physicians were able to adjust the acarbose dose for each patient as needed to minimize adverse effects. This dosing schedule is in contrast to clinical trials in which all patients received one specified dose of acarbose that was not titrated based on symptoms.[31]

Gastrointestinal Adverse Effects

Similar to metformin, the most commonly reported adverse effects with acarbose therapy pertain to the gastrointestinal tract. In a recent study, 84 percent of patients receiving acarbose therapy experienced gastrointestinal symptoms, compared to 38 percent of patients receiving placebo.[17] Flatulence, followed by diarrhea, have been the most commonly reported adverse effects in recent clinical trials.[5,6,17,21] Other common gastrointestinal symptoms include abdominal bloating, borborygmus, nausea, vomiting, and abdominal pain.[5,6,15,17,21,29] Fortunately, most of the adverse effects reported in clinical trials were considered to be mild or moderate.[29] These effects can largely be attributed to the actions of acarbose in the gastrointestinal tract. Because acarbose inhibits the alpha-glucosidase enzymes in the brush border of the small intestine, carbohydrates presenting to the brush border pass through undigested. Since the concentration of alpha-glucosidase enzymes is much lower in the distal portion of the small intestine, a large portion of undigested carbohydrates enters the large intestine. Fermentation of these carbohydrates leads to an increase in gas formation.[16,32]

Of particular note, acarbose is not expected to promote lactose intolerance. This expectation arises from the fact that the enzyme, lactase, responsible for the metabolism of lactose is a beta-glucosidase enzyme. Acarbose inhibits only alpha-amylase and alpha-glucosidase enzymes and has no activity on beta-glucosidase enzymes.[15] The selectivity of acarbose for alpha-glucosidase enzymes instead of beta-glucosidase enzymes limits the potential for the drug to provoke lactose intolerance.

One of the most successful methods to minimize gastrointestinal adverse effects seen with acarbose therapy is to initiate a low dose and slowly titrate upward. The recommended starting dose is 25 mg (1/2 of a 50 mg tablet) tid given with the first bite of a meal.[15] However, some clinicians suggest gastrointestinal effects may be further minimized by starting with 25 mg daily.[33] This therapy should be increased every four to eight weeks as tolerated to a maxi-

Table 1. Summary of select multicenter, randomized, double-blind, placebo-controlled trials reporting adverse effects to acarbose therapy in NIDDM patients

Reference	Daily dose (number of patients); duration of study	Number of patients on acarbose therapy	Gastrointestinal adverse effects (%)	Drop-out rate due to adverse events (%)	Comments
5	600 mg; 1 year	172	Flatulence 73.2, diarrhea 43.6, abdominal cramps/discomfort 25.0	19	No effect on liver function tests, no effect on vitamin or mineral levels, most adverse effects of mild to moderate intensity.
6	150–900 mg; Mean duration 151 days	104*	Flatulence 58, diarrhea 22, abdominal pain 18, dyspepsia 5, nausea 5	14	44 Patients (48%) received 900 mg; 4% and 9% of patients experienced increases in AST and ALT, respectively; 4 patients had transaminase elevations >1.8 ¥ ULN, all were asymptomatic, elevations reversed after discontinuation of therapy; 5 patients were reported to have decreased hemoglobin values.
27	900 mg; 24 weeks	103	Flatulence 76, diarrhea 33	NR	5% and 7% of patients experienced increases in AST and ALT, respectively; 3 patients had transaminase increases >3 ¥ ULN, all patients were asymptomatic, elevations were reversed on discontinuation of acarbose.
28	300 mg; 24 weeks	28	Flatulence 42.9, bloating 39.3	None	Small decreases in mean ALT, GGT, and uric acid were noted in the acarbose group.
17	600 mg; 24 weeks	143*	Flatulence 78.3, diarrhea 30.8, nausea 6.3, vomiting 4.2	11.9	Gastrointestinal adverse effects occurred in 83.9%, 4% and 5.9% experienced elevations in AST and ALT, respectively; 5 patients had transaminase elevations >3 ¥ ULN, all patients were asymptomatic, transaminase levels returned to normal upon discontinuation of therapy, 9% of patients had low serum uric acid levels.
19	300 (73), 600 (72), 900 (72) mg; 16 weeks	217*	Flatulence 81.4, diarrhea 34.6, nausea 5.1, abdominal pain 17.5	19	Incidence of gastrointestinal adverse effects were not dose related, five patients in the 600–900 mg treatment groups experienced elevations in serum transaminase levels, all patients were asymptomatic, and levels returned to normal upon discontinuation of therapy; headache reported in 12.4% of patients.

Note: AST = aspartate aminotransferase, ALT = alanine aminotransferase, ULN = upper limit of normal, NR = not reported, GGT = gamma-glutamyl transferase.
*Number of patients evaluated for adverse effects.

mum of 100 mg tid, or 50 mg tid for those patients weighing less than 60 kg.[15] Although conflicting data exist, there is some evidence to suggest the gastrointestinal effects seen with acarbose are dose related.[21,29] If these effects are dose related, a reduction in dose may alleviate some symptoms.[29] In clinical practice, dosage reduction is a viable option in those patients experiencing intolerable gastrointestinal symptoms.

Other ways to prevent further enhancement of these adverse effects is to limit the amount of sucrose intake and avoid administration of acarbose with other medications, such as cholestyramine and neomycin, that may induce the same type of symptoms.[4,32,34] There is some evidence to suggest that gastrointestinal effects may also be minimized by maintaining a diet high in complex carbohydrates with minimal intake of sucrose.[32,34,35] Sucrose, also known as cane sugar, is found in table sugar. Foods such as candy bars and baked sweets have a tendency toward considerable amounts of this sugar. Efforts to curb intake of sucrose-containing foods can therefore be a practical measure to minimize these adverse effects.

Gastrointestinal effects seen initially often subside with time.[16,36,37] In one particular study, 85 patients were randomized to receive acarbose 100 mg tid, glibenclamide, or placebo for 24 weeks. From Weeks 1 to 4, 37.5 percent of 28 patients receiving acarbose had complaints of flatulence, compared to 3.1 percent of the placebo group. By Weeks 9 to 12, only 9.4 percent of the acarbose group, compared to 0 percent of the placebo group, had the same complaints, and this number remained constant for the remainder of the 24-week evaluation period.[36] These data suggest tolerance to flatulence may develop following initiation of acarbose therapy. It is thought that this reduction in gastrointestinal effects may be caused by an induction of the alpha-glucosidase enzymes in the distal portion of the small intestine in response to an increased carbohydrate load.[16] Through this mechanism, less undigested carbohydrate is presented for fer-

mentation in the colon. To support this theory, a study evaluating the activity of sucrase, a member of the alpha-glucosidase enzyme family, in mice was conducted.[37] Diabetic and nondiabetic mice were divided into groups and fed normal diets or diets with varying doses of acarbose. Sucrase activity was measured in the proximal, middle, and distal regions of the small intestine. Acarbose eliminated the proximal to distal decline in sucrase activity in both diabetic and nondiabetic mice, as compared to the control mice. However, increases in middle and distal segment sucrase activity were much more pronounced in the diabetic mice than in the nondiabetic mice toward the end of the study period.[37] This evidence suggests sucrase activity may be induced by the presence of acarbose.

Elevated Hepatic Transaminases

In some clinical trials, elevated hepatic transaminases have been reported in patients receiving acarbose therapy.[6,17,21,30,36] There is some evidence to suggest these laboratory abnormalities are more common in patients receiving 600 mg daily or more of acarbose.[6,17,21,36] Elevations in aspartate aminotransferase and alanine aminotransferase were found to occur in up to 4 and 9 percent of acarbose patients in one study compared to 1 and 2 percent in the placebo group, respectively ($p = 0.368$ and $p = 0.10$).[6] Few patients have been reported to have values higher than three times the upper limit of normal.[17,30] Most of the patients who were reported to have aminotransferase elevations in the clinical trials were asymptomatic, and the abnormalities were rapidly reversed on discontinuation of acarbose.[6,17,21,29,30] It is important to note that many of the elevations were seen with doses of acarbose that are higher than the currently recommended maximum dose of 300 mg daily.[6,15,17,21,29] On further examination of data from clinical trials, it seems that certain patient populations may be predisposed to developing these abnormalities. These patient populations include females, African Americans, obese patients (body mass index greater than 29), and those patients who have been diagnosed with diabetes for more than five years.[29]

Due to the high number of elevated hepatic transaminase concentrations seen in clinical trials evaluating doses of 600 to 900 mg daily, the maximum recommended dose of acarbose is 300 mg daily.[4,6,17,21,30] If elevations in transaminase concentrations occur, a reduction in dose may be warranted. If laboratory elevations persist, acarbose therapy should be discontinued. Recommendations for transaminase monitoring include laboratory determinations at baseline and yearly or every three months in those patients receiving doses greater than 300 mg daily.[15]

Hypoglycemia

Acarbose is not likely to induce hypoglycemia in either the fasting or postprandial state due to its lack of effect on insulin release.[15] The incidence of hypoglycemia associated with acarbose has been reported to be equal to that of placebo.[29] Although the risk is low with monotherapy, acarbose may enhance the potential for hypoglycemic reactions in those patients receiving concomitant insulin or oral sulfonylureas due to its glucose-lowering actions.[4]

Due to the actions produced by acarbose on blood glucose concentrations, a reduction in insulin or oral sulfonylurea dosages may be warranted after initiation of acarbose therapy.[4,29] If hypoglycemia does develop during acarbose therapy, patients should not be treated with complex carbohydrates or foods containing sucrose. Instead, patients should be given products containing simple sugars, such as glucose tablets.

Due to the lack of inhibitory action on lactase, patients may also be given foods containing lactose, such as milk.

Anemia

A small percentage of patients receiving acarbose developed anemia in phase III American trials. Reductions in hemoglobin and hematocrit were seen in 1.1 percent of patients in the acarbose group, compared to 0.2 percent in the placebo group. It is thought that acarbose may limit iron absorption in the intestine. However, the Bayer International Clinical Data Pool did not reveal a higher incidence of anemia in patients treated with acarbose.[29]

Other

Hypocalcemia and reduced pyridoxine concentrations have been reported with acarbose therapy. However, these findings were not thought to be of clinical significance.[15]

• • •

Although there are a number of adverse effects associated with both metformin and acarbose therapy, these agents offer much-needed treatment options for the management of diabetes mellitus. In addition, a majority of these adverse effects are considered to be mild to moderate in severity and can be minimized or circumvented with proper education and management. To this end, medication compliance can be optimized to afford, in part, the best possible chance of managing diabetes mellitus with these novel antihyperglycemic agents.

REFRENCES

1. S.A. Eraker et al., "Understanding and Improving Patient Compliance," *Annals of Internal Medicine* 100 (1984): 258–268.
2. S.D. Sullivan et al., "Noncompliance with Medication Regimens and Subsequent Hospitalization: Literature Analysis and Cost of Hospitalization Estimate," *Journal*

of Research in Pharmaceutical Economics 2 (1990): 19–33.
3. L.E. Cluff, "Is Drug Toxicity a Problem of Great Magnitude? Yes!," in *Controversies in Therapeutics*, ed. L. Lasagna (Philadelphia: W.B. Saunders Company 1980), 44–50.

4. A.J. Krentz et al., "Comparative Tolerability Profiles of Oral Antidiabetic Agents," *Drug Safety* 11 (1994): 223–241.

5. J.L. Chiasson et al., "The Efficacy of Acarbose in the Treatment of Patients with Non–insulin-dependent Diabetes Mellitus. A Multicenter Controlled Clinical Trial," *Annals of Internal Medicine* 121 (1994): 928–935.

6. R.F. Coniff et al., "Long-term Efficacy and Safety of Acarbose in the Treatment of Obese Subjects with Non-insulin-dependent Diabetes Mellitus," *Archives of Internal Medicine* 154 (1994): 2,442–2,448.

7. R.A. DeFronzo et al., "Efficacy of Metformin in Patients with Non–insulin-dependent Diabetes Mellitus," *New England Journal of Medicine* 333 (1995): 541–549.

8. M.I. Harris et al., "Prevalence of Diabetes and Impaired Glucose Tolerance and Plasma Glucose Levels in U.S. Population Ages 20–74 yr," *Diabetes* 36 (1987): 523–534.

9. C.J. Bailey, "Biguanides and NIDDM," *Diabetes Care* 15 (1992): 755–772.

10. S.P. Clissold, and C. Edwards, "Acarbose: A Preliminary Review of Its Pharmacodynamic and Pharmacokinetic Properties, and Therapeutic Potential," *Drugs* 35 (1988): 214–243.

11. M. Nattrass, and K.G.M.M. "Biguanides," *Diabetologia* 14 (1978): 71–74.

12. M. Stumvoll et al., "Metabolic Effects of Metformin in Non–insulin-dependent Diabetes Mellitus," *New England Journal of Medicine* 333 (1995): 550–554.

13. C.J. Bailey, and M. Nattrass, "Treatment-Metformin," *Baillieres Clinical Endocrinology and Metabolism* 2 (1988): 455–476.

14. United Kingdom Prospective Diabetes Study Group, "United Kingdom Prospective Diabetes Study (UKPDS)13: Relative Efficacy of Randomly Allocated Diet, Sulphonylurea, Insulin, or Metformin in Patients with Newly Diagnosed Non-insulin-dependent Diabetes Followed for Three Years," *British Medical Journal* 310 (1995): 83–88.

15. Bayer Corporation, [Precose (acarbose) package insert]. (West Haven, CT: 1995).

16. H. Bischoff, "Pharmacology of Alpha-glucosidase Inhibition," *European Journal of Clinical Investigation* 24, no. 3 (1994): 3–10.

17. R.F. Coniff et al., "Multicenter, Placebo-controlled Trial Comparing Acarbose (Bay g 5421) with Placebo, Tolbutamide, and Tolbutamide-plus-acarbose in Non–insulin-dependent Diabetes Mellitus," *American Journal of Medicine* 98 (1995): 443–451.

18. Diabetes Control and Complications Trial Research Group, "The Effect of Intensive Treatment of Diabetes on the Development and Progression of Long-term Complications in Insulin-dependent Diabetes Mellitus," *New England Journal of Medicine* 329 (1993): 977–986.

19. American Diabetes Association, "Implications of the Diabetes Control and Complications Trial," *Diabetes Care* 19 (1995): S50–S52.

20. L.S. Hermann et al., "Therapeutic Comparison of Metformin and Sulfonylurea, Alone and in Various Combinations," *Diabetes Care* 17 (1994): 1,100–1,109.

21. R.F. Coniff et al., "Reduction of Glycosylated Hemoglobin and Postprandial Hyperglycemia by Acarbose in Patients with NIDDM," *Diabetes Care* 18 (1995): 817–824.

22. Bristol-Myers Squibb, [Metformin (Glucophage) package insert]. (Princeton, NJ: 1995).

23. P. Dandona et al., "Diarrhea and Metformin in a Diabetic Clinic," *Diabetes Care* 6 (1983): 472–474.

24. E. Haupt et al., "Oral Antidiabetic Combination Therapy with Sulfonylureas and Metformin," *Diabete & Metabolisme* 17 (1991): 224–231.

25. S.C. Gan, "Biguanide-associated Lactic Acidosis: Case Report and Review of the Literature," *Archives of Internal Medicine* 152 (1992): 2,333–2,336.

26. B.E. Wiholm, and M. Myrhed, "Metformin-associated Lactic Acidosis in Sweden 1977–91," *European Journal of Clinical Pharmacology* 44 (1993): 589–591.

27. N.S. Oates et al., "Influence of Oxidation Polymorphism on Phenformin Kinetics and Dynamics," *Clinical Pharmacology and Therapeutics* 34 (1983): 827–834.

28. C.J. Bailey, and R.C. Turner, "Metformin," *New England Journal of Medicine* 334 (1996): 574–579.

29. P. Hollander, "Safety Profile of Acarbose, an α-glucosidase Inhibitor," *Drugs* 44, no. 2 (1992): 47–53.

30. R.F. Coniff et al., "A Double-blind Placebo-controlled Trial Evaluating the Safety and Efficacy of Acarbose for the Treatment of Patients with Insulin-requiring Type II Diabetes," *Diabetes Care* 18 (1995): 928–932.

31. M. Spengler, and M. Cagatay, "The Use of Acarbose in the Primary-care Setting: Evaluation of Efficacy and Tolerability of Acarbose by Postmarketing Surveillance Study," *Clinical Investigative Medicine* 18 (1995): 325–331.

32. J.A. Balfour, and D. McTavish, "Acarbose: An Update of Its Pharmacology and Therapeutic Use in Diabetes Mellitus," *Drugs* 46 (1993): 1,025–1,054.

33. A.E. Martin, and P.A. Montgomery, "Acarbose: An α-glucosidase Inhibitor," *American Journal of Health-System Pharmacy* 53 (1996): 2,277–2,290.

34. D.J.A. Jenkins, and R.H. Taylor, "Acarbose: Dosage and Interaction with Sugars, Starch and Fibre," in *Proceedings of the First International Symposium on Acarbose, Montreux, October, 1981*, ed. W. Creutzfeldt (Amsterdam: Excerpta Medica, 1982), 86–96.

35. M. Toeller, "Nutritional Recommendations for Diabetic Patients and Treatment with α-glucosidase Inhibitors," *Drugs* 44, no. 3 (1992): 13–20.

36. J. Hoffmann, and M. Spengler, "Efficacy of 24-week Monotherapy with Acarbose, Glibenclamide, or Placebo in NIDDM Patients: The Essen Study," *Diabetes Care* 17 (1994): 561–566.

37. S.M. Lee et al., "The Effect of Alpha-glucosidase Inhibition on Intestinal Disaccharidase Activity in Normal and Diabetic Mice," *Metabolism* 32 (1983): 793–799.

PART III

Supportive Therapy and Treatment Concerns

Although hypoglycemic agents are the cornerstone of diabetes treatment, supportive care and supplementary diet and other treatment modalities are important components of care. Johnson and Beach develop a clear picture of the role of pharmacists in supporting and working with aspects of diabetes care not traditionally associated with drug therapy. This ever-evolving role in care of the diabetic patient is supported through direct patient interaction and education; a hallmark of pharmaceutical care. Patients with complicating disease states, such as hypertension, hyperlipidemia, and congestive heart failure, and the elderly patient present unique issues and require the development of strategies and care plans that support the achievement of the desired therapeutic objective. Chapters by Phillips and Ireland in this section address these complications and confounding therapeutic disease issues. This section culminates in a case study authored by Dr. Lenore Coleman that offers insight into a global and systematic approach to treatment.

CHAPTER 9

The Importance of the Pharmacist's Expanding Role on the Diabetes Team: Reinforcing Nutritional Guidelines for Improved Glycemic Control

Linda C. Johnson, RN, MS, CDE and Elizabeth Beach, MS, RD

The role of the pharmacist on the diabetes care team is expanding due to the increasing number of patients diagnosed with diabetes, limited health care dollars, and the education related to and required for patients by managed care organizations and insurance companies. In the past, training of patients in diabetes self-management skills has been inadequate, and this continues to be the case. Clinical pharmacists, in cooperation with physicians, have increased opportunities to provide education about medications and may include instructions for patients regarding the interaction of food consumed with changes in blood glucose levels. Because of monthly refills on prescribed medications, a patient's interaction with the pharmacist in the setting of a commercial pharmacy is more frequent than with any other member of the diabetes team. This contact offers an ideal educational opportunity. The action and efficacy of medications that affect the pancreas, hepatic glucose production, the utilization of glucose by muscle cells, and the absorption of glucose from the intestines are influenced directly by the meal plan. Nutritional guidelines, meal planning for the Type I and Type II patient, use of the exchange system, carbohydrate counting, artificial sweeteners, alcoholic beverages, and suggestions for guiding patients to establish eating habits that lead to improved diabetes control are important issues for every member of the diabetes team to address. The reinforcement of dietary principles may occur in the educational setting of the hospital or the clinic or within the commercial pharmacy setting. When the team presents accurate and current information, continuity of care and improved patient understanding are achieved. Key words: *diabetes control, diabetes education, diabetes management, dietitian, meal plan, pharmacist's role*

Diabetes is a complex disease that requires intensive treatment to prevent or delay the associated complications that develop due to poor control of blood glucose levels. New pathways of care and treatment algorithms give the physician guidelines for using a combination of therapies to offer the best treatment for the patient with Type I and Type II diabetes. The complexity of treatment regimens and the need for monitoring of the patient's progress require not only a physician but a team of dedicated health care professionals who assist patients in achieving success

in controlling their disease. The ideal diabetes care team is made up of the patient, a physician, a dietitian, a pharmacist, an exercise physiologist, a counselor, and a diabetes educator. A certified diabetes educator may be a nurse, physician, dietitian, pharmacist, or social worker.[1]

The concept of pharmaceutical care on the diabetes team involves more than the dispensing of medications. It has been defined as "the process through which a pharmacist cooperates with patients and other professionals in designing, implementing, and monitoring a therapeutic plan that will produce specific therapeutic outcomes for the patient."[2(p.533)] The pharmacist's role is taking on more importance as the frequency of care opportunities with the physician provided through managed care organizations is limited and the patient experiences changes in his or her insurance coverage. Patients may find they no longer have a continuing relationship with one physician. Rather, they may be forced to seek out medical care from a new physician and other health care providers.

The pharmacist has a significant impact on the outcome of the disease process by providing continuity of care and interaction with the patient in an ongoing educational intervention.[3] The pharmacist sees the patient in a variety of health care settings to include hospitals and clinics and, frequently, in the commercial setting for prescription refills. The pharmacist's role on the diabetes care team provides an excellent opportunity for education and reinforcement of principles taught by other team members. The pharmacist may be supportive and helpful and may have greater insight concerning the patient's family support system through observing interaction outside the medical office setting. The pharmacist can also provide information to other team members before the next scheduled physician appointment, intervening when a major medical crisis occurs. Patients may contact a pharmacist regarding an acute illness involving nausea and vomiting. This requires an immediate change in the nutritional needs of the patient. Guidelines for sick days become an essential part of the care plan and offer an occasion for collaboration between the pharmacist and the physician.

While meal planning is acknowledged as a cornerstone of intensive diabetes care, the actual teaching of guidelines for healthy nutrition has remained the responsibility of the registered dietitian on the diabetes care team. Unfortunately, patients are not always referred to a dietitian or nutritionist when the diagnosis of diabetes is made. Many times, only a printed meal plan is given to the patient along with an admonition to cut down on concentrated sweets and encouragement to lose weight. This seems to be the most common nutritional intervention during the early stages of Type II diabetes.[4] The patient is left on his or her own to figure out what to do about long-established eating habits and food addictions. Many patients already have a sense of guilt regarding their weight. They may even feel it is their own fault they have developed diabetes. After hearing the diagnosis of diabetes, while not surprised, most patients find themselves overwhelmed with the demands that are made for a changing lifestyle. Not only are they asked to make major changes in eating habits, exercise regimen, and general health habits, they may also be required to monitor blood glucose levels and record readings they do not understand. Patients find blood glucose monitoring helpful when they are able to incorporate blood glucose testing results into their care plan. With a minimal amount of instruction and a thorough explanation regarding the necessity for testing, the pharmacist is able to help patients master and value this new skill. Many find that while testing initially seems confining, it actually provides a tremendous sense of freedom and control.

THE DIABETES MEAL PLAN: RATIONALE

Nutritional therapy has been recognized as an essential component of care since the term *diabetes* was applied to this disease process in early Greek writing. This integral part of the treatment of diabetes, along with the importance of maintaining good nutrition while controlling blood glucose levels, has gone through a series of changes in the recommendations given to patients. From the early starvation diets that were thought to prolong life, to carbohydrate-restricted, high-fat meal plans, to the present recommendations that were published in 1994, the patient with diabetes needs to continue education regarding the latest information on good nutrition.

Appropriate meal planning, followed consistently, poses a great challenge for both the newly diagnosed and the long-term diabetes patient. Of the 5.8 million Americans with diabetes, 90 to 95 percent have Type II diabetes. Sixty to ninety percent of these people diagnosed with Type II diabetes are obese. Type II diabetes is most common after the age of 40, and these mature adults present with longstanding eating habits that may be difficult to change.[5] In America and most Western societies, food is viewed as a very important part of life. While many people strive to meet the challenge to be thin, actual food intake does not support that image. Many obese patients with diabetes greatly underestimate their total food intake. When questioned about food preferences and asked to recall patterns of food intake for the previous 24 hours and beyond, patients may begin to become aware of food addictions and unhealthy eating habits. When prompted to attach an emotion to intake of a particular food, they may realize that eating is often an emotional response to a given stimuli, resulting in unrecognized intake of excess calories. Learning food portion sizes and correct amounts of foods from various food groups rather than insisting patients follow strict diets may be the key to success in helping patients gain a sense of control of their eating habits and, ultimately, their glucose levels. Explaining the benefits of even minor weight loss (20 lbs. affect blood glucose levels significantly)[6] may motivate the patient to begin changing eating habits. The following educational concepts regarding the pathophysiology of Type II diabetes are suggestions for the pharmacist to use in helping patients understand what contributes to high blood glucose levels. Many patients express confusion over what causes blood glucose elevations and what physiological changes occur when they reduce their dietary intake.

Patients may be taught that there are three organs in the body that contribute to increased blood glucose levels:

1. *The pancreas:* In the patient with Type II diabetes, the pancreas may actually produce too much insulin in response to insulin resistance. There may be delayed or inadequate insulin release in some patients, while some patients are insulinopenic on diagnosis. (Insulin levels may be drawn upon diagnosis or when there is a diminished blood glucose control later in the course of the disease.) When patients re-duce their caloric intake, less insulin will be produced, and/or the insulin produced will become more effective.

2. *The liver:* Glucose production and release of glucose from the liver of the patient with Type II diabetes are increased. Hepatic glucose production is decreased with weight loss.

3. *The muscles (peripheral tissues):* A primary defect in Type II diabetes is insulin resistance at the receptor site resulting in diminished tissue sensitivity to insulin. Peripheral glucose uptake (explained to the patient as uptake from muscle tissue) is enhanced when the patient reduces caloric intake and loses weight.

One pound of body fat contains approximately 3,500 kcal. Eating 500 to 1,000 calories/day less than a usual intake or less than maintenance calorie needs should result in a weight loss of 1 to 2 lb. per week. The recommended caloric intake level per day is no less than 1,200 calories for women and 1,600 calories for men to ensure that the meal plan includes adequate vitamins, minerals, nutrients, and energy for the ambulatory patient.

As patients reduce caloric intake, blood glucose levels will begin to decrease even before any appreciable weight loss is noticed. When the patient refills or receives a new prescription, the pharmacist can explain that medication dosage may need to be adjusted as the patient loses weight and recognizes patterns of lowered blood glucose through self-monitoring test results. The pharmacist should encourage good communication between the patient and the physician in this matter.

THE GOALS OF MEDICAL NUTRITION THERAPY*

The following sections on the goals of Medical Nutrition Therapy, Nutrition for Patients

*Source: Adapted from "Nutrition Recommendations and Principles for People with Diabetes Mellitus," Position Statement, Journal of Clinical Applied Nutrition Research Education, Vol. 20, Supplement, *Diabetic Care,* January 1997.

with Type I and Type II Diabetes, An Overview of Nutritional Components are summarized in part from the American Diabetes Association position statement.

- maintenance of near-normal blood glucose levels through balance of food intake and/or insulin (either exogenous or endogenous) and/or oral hypoglycemic agents as required
- achievement and maintenance of optimal serum lipid levels
- sufficient calories to achieve and maintain reasonable body weight and adequate calorie intake to ensure normal growth and development for the juvenile with Type I diabetes
- treatment and intervention for the acute complications of diabetes that may be related to nutritional intervention: hypoglycemia, short-term illness, changes in blood glucose due to exercise, stress, either physical or emotional, glucose toxicity (an immodulator of beta cell function), and maintenance of blood pressure less than 135/85 mm Hg if the patient is hypertensive[4]
- improvement of overall health through optimal nutrition
- functional, individualized meal planning that works within both the individual and family lifestyle, resulting in improved patient emotional well-being and long-term empowerment so that the patient may adhere to suggested treatment modalities

The principles of meal planning for Type I and Type II diabetes are similar, but there are definite differences in the recommendations made to patients. These differences involve the age of the patient; the duration of the disease; the pharmaceutical treatment plan; other disease processes; the patient's willingness to follow a prescribed meal plan; and, as diabetes progresses, the presence of hypoglycemia unawareness. It is important for the health care professional to remember that a patient's compliance with any suggestion for change will be related to the patient's perception of the seriousness of his or her diabetes.

Patients with Type II diabetes who are told they have "borderline diabetes" or who are advised simply to cut back on concentrated sweets without the benefit of counseling with a registered dietitian will be much more resistant to making changes suggested by other members of the diabetes care team. Patients with Type I diabetes who are diagnosed as children will probably go through rebellion to the meal plan during adolescence due to peer pressure and other social demands. Support from the family, physician, dietitian, and diabetes educator and intervention by a counselor may help the teenager get back on track in controlling his or her disease. Most teenagers do not respond to discussions related to the possible complications of allowing blood glucose levels to be uncontrolled over an extended period of time. However, most are receptive to changes that make living in the "here and now" more tolerable. Small, simple blood glucose monitors, insulin injection devices (prefilled syringes, pens with cartridges), or an insulin pump that allows more flexibility in the timing of meals and snacks are ideas that may help adolescents follow their diabetes management plan. Suggestions for making adjustments in insulin doses to accommodate social functions reassure adolescents that they can control their own disease while still enjoying life with their friends.

Nutrition Therapy For The Patient With Type I Diabetes

- Integrate insulin with eating and exercise habits.
- With conventional therapy, synchronize food with insulin, follow a consistent meal plan, and make adjustments in the insulin dose according to preprandial blood glucose levels.
- With intensive therapy, integrate insulin into the lifestyle, and make adjustments in insulin dosage to compensate for lifestyle changes. Patients may be taught to make anticipatory

adjustments in insulin doses prior to meals. This therapy usually includes carbohydrate counting and adjustments for planned exercise. Intensive therapy includes insulin infusion pumps or multiple injections using Regular/Hummalog insulin as boluses before meals and an intermediate insulin, NPH or Lente, or long-acting insulin, Ultra Lente, used as a basal insulin dose.[7]

Nutrition Therapy for the Patient with Type II Diabetes

- Stress the importance of controlling lipid levels as well as blood glucose.
- Restrict calories for consistent, moderate weight loss and weight maintenance.
- Place patient on a meal plan rather than a diet for long-term control of diabetes. Offer education to help patients make better food choices, modify fat intake, restrict alcohol intake, and reduce sodium intake (indicated in patients who are sensitive to sodium).
- Increase physical activity along with meal planning (enhances effectiveness of endogenous insulin, reduces insulin resistance).[8]

OVERVIEW OF NUTRITIONAL COMPONENTS

An overview of the nutritional components relevant to successful meal planning for the patient with diabetes includes the following.

Calories

Calories should be sufficient to achieve and maintain a reasonable body weight.

Carbohydrate

Carbohydrate percentages and types may vary, but the most current recommendations suggest that approximately 50 to 60 percent of daily calories should come from carbohydrate sources. The amount of carbohydrate for the patient is based on individualized eating habits, glucose, and lipid goals. Emphasis is on the total amount of carbohydrate versus the type of carbohydrate eaten and on the spacing of carbohydrate intake throughout the day. Patients must be cautioned regarding skipping or severely reducing carbohydrate intake at one meal and overindulging at the next meal. Modest amounts of sucrose and other refined sugars may be acceptable, contingent on metabolic control and body weight. Recent studies indicate that fruit and milk have lower glycemic response than most starches, and sucrose produces a glycemic response similar to that of bread, rice, and potatoes. Various starches have different glycemic responses. Emphasis should be placed on the importance of ingesting consistent amounts of carbohydrates at the same time daily. The source is less important than the total amount.

Protein

The exact ideal percentage of dietary protein is still undetermined, but 10 to 20 percent of total daily calories is usually recommended for patients with diabetes. This may be from animal or vegetable sources. The recommended allowance for patients experiencing the evidence of diabetes-related nephropathy is 0.8 percent g/kg body weight or approximately 10 percent of total daily calories. This appears to be sufficiently restrictive in most instances. Once the glomerular filtration rate begins to fall, further restriction may prove useful in selected patients. There is concern that nutritional deficiency of protein may occur in some individuals and may be associated with muscle weakness. Meal plans that restrict protein should be individually designed by registered dietitians familiar with these problems.

Fat

Ideally, the patient with diabetes will consume less than 30 percent of total daily calories from fat. This is also the recommendation found in the *Dietary Guidelines for Americans*. This allowance provides for normal growth and development in children and adolescents. If obesity and weight loss are the primary issues, then dietary fat reduction is an efficient way to reduce caloric intake, although fat restriction is not usually recommended in children under two years of age. It is recommended that less than 10 percent of total fat come from saturated fats. When patients with diabetes present with elevated low-density lipoprotein (LDL) as a primary, continuing problem, the *National Cholesterol Education Program Step II* diet guidelines include: reducing total saturated fat to less than 7 percent, with less than 30 percent of daily calories from fat and less than 200 mg/day dietary cholesterol. If elevated triglycerides and very–low-density lipoproteins are the primary problems, weight loss, exercise, and a moderate increase in monounsaturated fat intake are encouraged. Recommendations include: less than 10 percent of calories from saturated and polyunsaturated fats, monounsaturated fats up to 20 percent of calories, and a more moderate intake of carbohydrates. In obese patients, any increase in fat may make weight loss more difficult. Patients with triglycerides greater than 300 mg/dL will require a reduction of all types of dietary fat, pharmaceutical intervention; and careful monitoring of glycemic levels, lipid status, and body weight. Assessment of nutrition status and eating habits by a registered dietitian is essential.

Fiber

Fiber recommendations for the diabetic patient are the same as those for the general public, approximately 20 to 35 g/day. Fiber is filling, and many patients find it helps them feel more satisfied as they reduce total caloric intake. Some soluble fibers may delay the absorption of carbohydrates from the small intestine and have a minor effect on glycemic control. This effect may need to be taken into account by the patient on intensive insulin therapy who has frequent intake of high-fiber foods and who uses carbohydrate counting to enhance glycemic control. Total fiber intake may also need to be modified for patients experiencing gastric paresis, a delayed emptying of the stomach causing wide fluctuations in glycemic levels.

Alternative Sweeteners

Dietary fructose causes a slower, smaller rise in blood glucose than sucrose and some starchy sources of carbohydrates. However, large amounts of fructose can have an adverse effect on blood lipids. Naturally occurring fructose in fruits and vegetables need not be restricted so long as portion sizes are consistent and weight is reduced or maintained. The nonnutritive sweeteners saccharin, aspartame, and acesulfame K are all approved for use by the Food and Drug Administration.

Sodium

Avoid excessive amounts (greater than 400 mg/single serving, greater than 1,000 mg/meal) in patients who are sensitive to the effects of sodium. Patients should be reminded that sodium is present not only in salt but in a wide variety of food additives, fast foods, and convenience food items.

Alcohol

Alcohol may be used in moderate amounts when diabetes is well controlled. Concerns include hypoglycemia, excessive calories, triglyceride elevation, and possible abuse of alcohol. Patients who use insulin or sulfonylurea drugs should limit alcohol intake to two drinks per day and be reminded to consume alcohol only in conjunction with meals.

Micronutrients

Provided the meal plan is adequate and a patient has no malabsorption problems or chewing and/or swallowing difficulties, there is no need for vitamin or mineral supplementation.[9]

Other Foods

Patients may have questions concerning the plethora of "diet" foods or candies that have recently appeared on both pharmacy and grocery store shelves. Patients should be cautioned that not all "diet" foods are acceptable and that even these foods must be worked into their meal plan. Many fat-free foods are actually higher in sugar and total carbohydrate than the original food items they replace. These foods may not be appropriate for the diabetic meal plan. Most are certainly not to be considered as "free foods." As a general rule of thumb, the portion size containing approximately 10 to 15 g of carbohydrate may occasionally be worked into the meal plan as a fruit or bread serving.

The Role of Pharmacists and Others

Ideally, the pharmacist and other health care professionals on the diabetes care team will reinforce the nutrition teaching that is done by the registered dietitian or nutritionist. However, evidence exists that many patients with diabetes are not seen by a dietitian early in their disease process. Many patients are not referred until they are placed on insulin therapy. For optimum diabetes control, patients should experience early nutrition intervention in the form of assessment and counseling by an experienced nutrition professional. Ideally, this should take place as soon as the diagnosis of diabetes or impaired glucose tolerance is made.

While the United States is flooded with "diet advice," weight charts, and "quick fixes" for losing weight, the general population is also heavier, and the incidence of diabetes is increasing at an alarming rate. In some commercial pharmacy settings, clinics, or hospitals, pharmacists are a source of information regarding the use of over-the-counter diet aids and prescription medications for weight loss and obesity. These medications need to be administered accompanied by information about the diabetes meal plan and/or healthy nutrition. For the patient with diabetes who questions the pharmacist regarding improving glycemic control, nutritional counseling with a registered dietitian or nutritionist must be the first suggestion considered.

MEAL-PLANNING APPROACHES

When a patient is first made aware of a problem with glucose control and/or diabetes, the first questions asked usually concern what he or she will be allowed to eat. After a brief assessment of the patient's present eating habits, the health care professional can encourage the patient to begin making changes by simply cutting down on the amount of concentrated sweets and fats in the diet and reducing the portion sizes of the food consumed. Most patients respond well to simple instructions. A 3 oz. serving of meat is approximately the size of the palm of the hand, while a cup of starch, two starch servings, or two carbohydrates (rice, noodles, potatoes) are the size of a patient's fist. An ounce of cheese is about the size of the thumb. Although the size of a patient's hand may vary, this simplistic approach is an idea patients can begin to use immediately in the early stages of nutrition therapy. Basic nutrition guidelines include healthy food choices, the food-guide pyramid, and perhaps sample menus that offer food choice suggestions for the patient. The food pyramid offers a visual guideline for patients, encouraging the consumption of grains, vegetables, and fruits, while suggesting the reduction of fat and sugar intake. For the patient who may appear overwhelmed with making food choices, frozen low-fat, low-calorie meals offer an alternative that may help during this time.

As the education process begins, the exchange system is introduced to help the patient grasp an understanding of food groups and portion sizes. *The Revised Exchange Lists for Meal Planning* includes important changes. The meat group now has four lists rather than three. Very lean meat is a new exchange suggesting the use of white-fleshed fish and white-meat turkey or chicken. The fat group is divided into monounsaturated, polyunsaturated, and saturated fats, allowing the educator to make recommendations regarding "healthy fats." The carbohydrate group lists starch, fruit, and milk and "other carbohydrates" with 12 to 15 g/serving, allowing the patient to interchange servings and add flexibility to the meal plan.

The exchange lists allow patients to use portion control versus calorie counting, which may be viewed by many as either too time consuming or confusing. Asking a patient to keep a food diary in the early stages of nutritional counseling gives an account of the amount of food consumed and the time the food was eaten. This information, along with blood glucose testing results and the schedule for insulin and medications, allows the clinician to adjust meal-planning guidelines and the dosage of medications. By evaluating weight loss/maintenance and the results of the hemoglobin A1c, a patient's progress and level of control may be monitored.

CARBOHYDRATE COUNTING

As the patient gains understanding of the basics of nutrition, carbohydrate counting and fat counting will give the patient greater flexibility in making food choices. This theory assumes that the carbohydrates in foods, found in starch, fruit, and milk, directly affect the postprandial blood glucose rise. It is estimated that 90 percent of carbohydrate is converted to glucose within one to two hours after it is consumed. With carbohydrate counting, the patient is asked to look at the total carbohydrate eaten rather than the source of the carbohydrate. With this understanding, the patient can strive for consistency in the total amount of carbohydrate used at each meal. Although this may suggest that the patient will have freedom to indulge in concentrated sweets at will, the nutritionist/dietitian stresses the importance of healthy food choices daily. There will be provisions made for occasional use of high-sugar foods. Patients, who become proficient in carbohydrate-counting quickly become cognizant of what causes dramatic rises in their blood glucose levels.[10]

The "Glycemic Index" (GI), popular several years ago, is once again being considered as a valuable tool for patients with diabetes. The GI ranks foods based on their immediate effects on blood glucose levels, looking at the two- to three-hour postprandial rise in glucose. A new book, *The G.I. Factor: The Glycaemic Index Solution,* takes a definitive look at this tool for a second time. Foods are ranked as having a high GI if the effect of eating a portion will cause a rapid, high rise in blood glucose levels. Glucose

is rated at 100, followed by instant rice, white rice, and baked potato. Foods having a low GI are ranked between 14 and 33, and include beans; barley; peanuts; and low-fat, artificially sweetened yogurt. These foods may produce a slower rise in the glucose plasma value.

While patients may find the concepts in this book interesting, it becomes apparent to most patients that they must have an individualized GI that they discover for themselves.[11] It is also essential for patients to consider what they consume with the carbohydrates and how protein and fat affect the absorption of glucose from the gut. When carbohydrates are eaten by themselves, there is a greater rise in blood glucose than when some protein and fat are consumed in the context of a meal. The meal is also more satisfying when small amounts of fat and protein are eaten, and this helps to prevent overeating between meals. The blood glucose may stay more consistent, without the exaggerated "peaks" due to excess carbohydrate intake. Consistency both in carbohydrate level and caloric intake, and proper meal spacing throughout the day, are essential for good control of blood glucose levels.

OTHER SOURCES OF CARBOHYDRATES

Patients have many questions about concentrated sweets as part of the meal plan. In the past, sucrose and other sugars were severely restricted for the patient with diabetes. However, studies have shown that limited sucrose can become part of a healthy meal plan and does not impair blood glucose control in either Type I or Type II diabetes. Sucrose needs to be counted as part of the total carbohydrate for any meal. Sucrose consumed by itself will have more of an effect on blood glucose levels than when it is consumed as part of a meal. Fructose has been shown to produce a smaller rise in plasma glucose than isocaloric amounts of sucrose and most starchy carbohydrates. Large amounts of fructose may have an adverse effect on serum cholesterol and LDL cholesterol and, for this reason, may not be advantageous to incorporate as a sweetening agent.

Naturally occurring fructose in fruits and vegetables need not be avoided by patients with dyslipidemia. Sorbitol, mannitol, and xylitol are sugar alcohols that produce a lower glycemic response than glucose, sucrose, or other nutritive sweeteners. However, an excessive amount of sugar alcohol can cause diarrhea and intestinal discomfort.

THE ROLE OF PROTEIN IN THE DIABETIC MEAL PLAN

Although the exact amount of protein needed by patients with diabetes has not been determined, the role of protein is very important. Protein, from both animal and vegetable sources, is broken down in the intestines into amino acids. These are used by the body to repair tissues and to form new tissue. In the blood stream, both amino acids and glucose stimulate the release of insulin. Insulin then enhances muscle amino acid uptake and stimulates muscle protein synthesis. Children who are in poor diabetes control and receive inadequate insulin do not have comparable growth rates with nondiabetic children. Adults who have inadequate insulin, either endogenous or exogenous, may experience difficulty with wound healing. Questions still remain concerning protein intake in the diabetes meal plan, but current recommendations include 10 to 20 percent of total calories from protein sources.

A new bestseller, *Enter the Zone*,[12] has sold more than a million copies and is considered one of the latest diet crazes in America. It suggests that consuming too many carbohydrates may lead to hyperinsulinemia, weight gain, heart disease, and diabetes. It recommends greater levels of protein intake than are necessary to maintain good health for any individual but especially for those individuals diagnosed with diabetes.

The theories in this book are not based on any published clinical studies, and the advice is in contrast to that given by most nutrition researchers and dietitians who have determined that the average American diet probably contains twice the amount of protein required. There does not appear to be a protein deficiency in our society except perhaps in the older, compromised population who may require more protein than the suggested 10 to 20 percent of total calories.[13] In addition, the animal protein sources most often selected by Americans contain more saturated fat than is desirable.[13]

The protein recommendations in this and other diet books touting high-protein, low-carbohydrate eating are not based on sound nutritional principles. For a nation already suffering the high incidence of cardiovascular disease that is present in the United States, recommending high levels of protein, with the resultant high intake of saturated fat, would seem to be ill advised. For diabetic patients who are already at greatly increased risk for the development of both cardiovascular and kidney diseases, such recommendations would be far worse. In meal planning for the patient with diabetes, food preferences, blood glucose levels, type and amount of glucose-lowering medication prescribed, and other factors must be taken into consideration. Individuals differ in their needs. For example, patients receiving insulin and high doses of oral glucose-lowering agents (sulfonylureas) may feel hungry between meals if sufficient protein is not included in the meal plan. Patients receiving insulin also may require a protein-containing snack prior to bedtime to reduce the likelihood of dangerous hypoglycemic episodes during the night. This may be especially problematic for the patient who takes an intermediate acting insulin at supper time. The patient with gestational diabetes often requires a higher protein and fat intake at breakfast to reduce glucose levels resulting from the glucose intolerance often seen in the early morning hours. Additional carbohydrate intake may be tolerated later in the day. For optimal success, patients should have access to individualized meal plans that meet their specific needs and correlate with their lifestyle and personal food preferences.

FAT CONSUMPTION FOR THE PATIENT WITH DIABETES

The decade of the 1990s could well be called "the fat-free decade of the 20th century," or so Americans would like to believe. Not only are there more fat-free products on the shelves of every grocery store, but that missing fat seems to have been transferred to the American physique. The average American, heavier than the last generation while claiming to eat less fat, is, in reality, eating as much as a decade ago and accompanying the fat with more carbohydrates. While most Americans eat far more fat than is either necessary or desirable, fat is valuable in the diabetic meal plan and should be included as part of a healthy diet. But how much is enough?

Fat is an enjoyable and healthy component of good nutrition for individuals who have normal lipid levels and who maintain desirable weight levels. Indeed, fat is necessary for normal growth and development in children and adolescents, and it is important for all individuals as a source of essential fatty acids and a carrier of fat-soluble vitamins. Fat slows digestion and aids satiety by "turning off the hunger switch." It certainly adds to the personal enjoyment of foods. Therefore, it is important that fat be included in all meal plans. Even patients with elevated lipid levels require some fat in their meal plans, although guidelines for fat consumption in these individuals include reducing overall fat intake to less than 30 percent of daily calories with less than 7 to 10 percent in the form of saturated fats. However, individuals with genetic predisposition to intractable lipid elevation may require lipid-lowering medication in conjunction with fat restriction to achieve satisfactory disease outcome.

As with other nutritional components, the recommended amount and distribution of fat calories vary and should be individualized based on nutritional assessment and treatment goals. Weight-loss goals, lipid levels, individual patient eating habits, and motivation levels are the factors to be considered when determining recommended fat intake.[14]

VITAMINS, MINERALS, AND CHROMIUM

Vitamin and mineral supplementation recommendations vary from physician to physician. When patients are in good general health and dietary intake is adequate, there is little need for additional vitamin and mineral supplements. However, when a patient is newly diagnosed and is attempting to make major lifestyle changes under the emotional stress of the diagnosis, nutritional intake may become overly regimented or inadequate. For this reason, many patients with diabetes are advised to take a daily vitamin supplement containing approximately 100 percent of the recommended daily allowances (RDA). Antioxidant vitamins may also be prescribed, although this therapy is controversial. There are still many questions about the role of magnesium deficiency in insulin resistance, carbohydrate intolerance, and hypertension. Available data suggest that evaluation of magnesium level is done only in patients who show signs of hypomagnesia.[15]

Chromium and diabetes are frequently mentioned together, and more questions are asked about this supplement. Chromium by itself is poorly absorbed; therefore, supplements are usually combined with picolinic acid to enhance the absorption of the mineral. Chromium only lowers blood glucose levels when insulin is present. The mechanism appears to be that chromium binds insulin to the cell membrane. However, at this time, there is no reliable way to determine if chromium deficiency is present. The response to chromium depends largely on the degree of glucose intolerance. Chromium is a nutritional supplement and should not be seen as a pharmacological intervention for diabetes. Claims that chromium can cure diabetes are false and misleading and give the diabetic population unfounded hope. Some individuals who have shown benefit from supplementation with chromium are those who have impaired glucose tolerance. If chromium deficiency is considered a possible causative factor for individuals presenting with slight elevations in blood glucose or lipid levels, a trial of chromium supplements may be warranted. A safe and adequate amount of chromium is 50 to 200 mcg/day.[16]

•   •   •

Each member of the diabetes care team has a role in helping patients achieve blood glucose control through meal planning, monitoring, and medications. While the role of each team member focuses on a specific aspect of care, it is important that the team work as a unit reinforcing the principles of control and giving information that is current and accurate. Each patient has unique and individualized needs that are addressed by the responsible team member for that aspect of care. Pharmacists may aid in the reinforcement of dietary principles by answering patient questions; encouraging limited fat intake and gradual weight loss where warranted; and stressing the simple but effective principles of consistent food intake, appropriately spaced, throughout the day. The very complex and changing nature of diabetes demands more than one physician to provide the best care for the patient. Patients need a team of specialists to assist them in understanding basic principles of control so that they win not only a life that is longer, but a life of quality and good health.

REFERENCES

1. C. Kilo, and L.J. Johnson, *Diabetes Model for Care* (1996).

2. C.D. Hepler, and L.M. Strand, "Opportunities and Responsibilities in Pharmaceutical Care," *American Journal of Hospital Pharmacy* 47 (1990): 533–542.

3. M.K. Van Veldhuizen-Scott et al., "Developing and Implementing a Pharmaceutical Care Model in an Ambulatory Setting for Patients with Diabetes," *The Diabetes Educator* 21, no. 2 (1995): 117–123.

4. D.L. Lorber, "Nutrition Guidelines for People with Diabetes," *Practical Diabetology* 15, no. 1 (1996): 9–15.

5. American Diabetes Association, *Diabetes 1996: Vital Statistics* (Alexandria, Va.: American Diabetes Association, 1996), 3.

6. A. Daly, "Nutrition Management," in *Therapy for Diabetes Mellitus and Related Disorders,* 2nd ed., ed. H. Leibowitz (Alexandria, Va.: American Diabetes Association, 1994), 95–101.

7. M.A. Sperling, "Nutrition," in *Medical Management of Insulin-dependent (Type I) Diabetes,* 2nd ed. (Alexandria, Va.: American Diabetes Association, 1994), 57–58.

8. H. Rifkin and H. Leibowitz, et al., "Nutrition," in *Medical Management of Non–insulin-dependent (Type II) Diabetes,* 3rd ed. (Alexandria, Va.: American Diabetes Association, 1994), 28–34.

9. American Diabetes Association, "Clinical Practice Recommendations, 1997," *The Journal of Clinical and Applied Research and Education* 20, no. 1 (1997): S14–S17.

10. A. Daly, "Carbohydrate Counting: New Teaching Resources," *Practical Diabetology* 15, no. 1 (1996): 19–23.

11. R. Mendosa, "What Exactly Will Happen if I Eat This Bran Muffin? The Glycemic Index Can Tell You," *Diabetes Interview* 49 (August 1996): 1, 9, 12.

12. B. Sears, and W. Lawren, *Enter the Zone* (Regan Books, 1995), 77–80.

13. B. Liebman, "Carbo-Phobia: Zoning Out on the New Diet Books," *Nutrition Action Health Letter* 23, no. 6 (1996): 3–5.

14. *Maximizing the Role of Nutrition in Diabetes Management* [highlights of a clinical education program] (Alexandria, Va.: American Diabetes Association, 1994), 30–31.

15. A.D. Mooradian et al., "Selected Vitamins and Minerals in Diabetes," *Diabetes Care* 17 (Alexandria, Va.: American Diabetes Association, 1994): 464–479.

16. R.A. Anderson et al., "Supplemental Chromium Effects on Glucose, Insulin, Glucagon, and Urinary Chromium Losses in Subjects Consuming Controlled Low-Chromium Diets," *American Journal of Clinical Nutrition* 54 (1991): 909–916.

CHAPTER 10

Treatment of Hypertension in Patients with Diabetes

Bradley G. Phillips, PharmD

Approximately 3 million Americans have the dual diagnosis of hypertension and diabetes. Both conditions are associated with and are risk factors for cardiovascular events, nephropathy, and retinopathy. When these conditions coexist, the prevalence, progression, and severity of these adverse outcomes are dramatically enhanced. For these reasons, hypertension should be treated aggressively and early in the diabetic patient to curtail the morbidity and mortality associated with these disease states. To this end, a number of consensus statements have been formulated and promulgated in an effort to increase the awareness of this condition and to provide guidelines by which optimal care may be afforded to patients. In addition, specific patient and drug-related factors and conditions should be considered so patients can be committed to the optimal therapeutic plan. The outcome to attain optimal blood pressure should be mirrored by efforts to obtain glycemic and lipidemic control. By the implementation and optimization of effective therapeutic measures, which have the least amount of impact on the patient's concomitant disease states and body chemistry, positive differences in outcomes may be realized in this population. Key words: *diabetes, drug therapy, hypertension*

Approximately three million Americans have both hypertension and diabetes.[1,2] For patients with non–insulin dependent diabetes mellitus (NIDDM), the incidence of essential hypertension increases with age and exists in about one out of every two patients.[2,3] In patients with both insulin-dependent diabetes mellitus (IDDM) and NIDDM, diabetic nephropathy is also an important factor for the development of hypertension.[4] Uncontrolled hypertension and diabetes are risk factors for cardiovascular mortality and morbidity, renal dysfunction, and retinopathy.[5,6] In patients with diabetes, the presence of hypertension may lead to premature and more severe cardiovascular events as well as perpetuate renal and retinal dysfunction. The relationship between diabetes and hypertension is not fully understood, but it is clear that these diseases are interrelated.[3] Hyperinsulinemia (insulin resistance) may affect the sympathetic and renin-angiotensin systems sodium excretion by the kidneys and interfere with peripheral vasodilation.[7–9] These effects may contribute, in part, to elevations in blood pressure. Furthermore, hyperinsulinemia may contribute to or is associated with dyslipidemia and obesity.[10] Although the exact interrelation between hypertension and diabetes is unknown, patients with both conditions are at increased risk for associated morbidity and mortality than with either hypertension or diabetes alone. For these reasons, patients with hypertension and diabetes should be treated early and aggressively.[3] To accomplish this goal, a number of consensus statements on the management and treatment of hypertension and diabetes have been developed and promulgated.[3,11,12,13]

CONSENSUS STATEMENTS

A number of expert panels and government agencies have offered consensus statements with respect to the detection, management, and treatment of hypertension and diabetes. To this end, the goal of these efforts, in general, is to increase awareness of the impact of hypertension and diabetes as well as guide health care providers to provide optimal care for patients with diabetes and hypertension. For example, The National High Blood Pressure Education Program Working Group has published and updated its report on diabetes and hypertension.[3,14] As part of this publication, a treatment algorithm is offered to outline an approach to the management of patients with hypertension and diabetes (see Figure 1).

As depicted in the algorithm (Figure 1), the goal of therapy and the treatment for hypertension in the diabetic patient are outlined. The goal blood pressure to be attained in hypertensive diabetic patients is less than 130/85 mm Hg. To achieve this goal, nondrug therapies and lifestyle modifications should be employed for three months. If an inadequate response or considerable progress has not been achieved, drug therapy should be initiated. Drugs from various classes that include angiotensin converting enzyme (ACE) inhibitors, alpha blockers, calcium channel antagonists, and low-dose diuretics may be initially considered while continuing nondrug and lifestyle modification efforts. Due to the compelling and growing evidence for the renal protective effects of ACE inhibitors, they are now considered the drugs of choice in insulin-dependent and non–insulin-dependent diabetic patients who have albuminuria or proteinuria. If initial monotherapy with any of the above agents does not provide an adequate response, the dose may be increased, another agent may be tried, or a second agent may be added to the therapy. Failing this, a second or third antihypertensive agent may be added to attain the desired blood pressure. If not prescribed for initial therapy, low-dose diuretic therapy should be included in subsequent therapy. Beta blockers, although effective in controlling blood pressure, are reserved for those hypertensive diabetic patients who have a clear indication other than hyperten-

sion for beta-blocker therapy. This treatment algorithm outlines general treatment strategies that should be considered along with other patient and drug-related issues and considerations before a specific treatment plan is formulated for each diabetic patient.[14]

THERAPY CONSIDERATIONS

Selection of the optimal antihypertensive agent in each patient with diabetes should be based on the agent's impact on morbidity and mortality, glucose, electrolytes, insulin resistance, and lipids, as well as the cost of therapy and associated drug-induced adverse effects. Thiazide diuretics and beta blockers have been shown to reduce cardiovascular morbidity and mortality in patients with hypertension.[15–18] For these reasons, they are considered the initial drugs of choice in the treatment of hypertension by the Joint National Committee on the Detection, Evaluation, and Treatment of High Blood Pressure (JNC).[19] However, no study to date has evaluated the impact of these agents, or others, on cardiovascular morbidity and mortality in the diabetic population. It is assumed that diuretics and beta blockers will indeed confer the same beneficial effect on morbidity and mortality in hypertensive diabetic patients as they do in nondiabetic patients. There are several studies to give support to or possibly refute this presumption. The Systolic Hypertension in the Elderly Program (SHEP) evaluated the efficacy of low-dose diuretic, with atenolol and reserpine if needed, with placebo in 4,736 patients with an average baseline systolic blood pressure of 160 mm Hg or greater and a diastolic blood pressure of less than 90 mm Hg.[20] The study found that with an average of four and a half years of active treatment, there was a 36 and 27 percent decrease in fatal and nonfatal strokes and myocardial infarctions, respectively, compared to those patients receiving placebo. A subsequent analysis to compare study outcomes in patients with NIDDM to patients without diabetes enrolled in SHEP revealed that both groups had a 34 percent reduction in cardiovascular disease rate at five years.[21] Further, the absolute risk reduction for treatment compared to placebo in

Treatment Goal < 130/85 mm Hg.

Lifestyle Modifications
- Regular aerobic physical activity
- Reduction in sodium intake
- Smoking cessation
- Dietary intervention to control hyperglycemia and dyslipidemia
- Weight reduction
- Moderation of alcohol intake

(monitor and appropriately treat associated dyslipidemias)

Inadequate Response* (after 3 months)

Continue Lifestyle Modifications plus . . .
Initiate Pharmacologic Selection (in alphabetical order)

ACE inhibitors, alpha blockers, calcium antagonists, and diuretics in low dose are preferred because of fewer adverse effects on glucose homeostasis, lipid profile, and renal function

(ACE inhibitors are drugs of choice in patients with albuminuria/proteinuria)

(Beta blockers can adversely affect peripheral blood flow, prolong hypoglycemia, and mask hypoglycemic symptoms)

Inadequate Response*

| Increase drug dose | Substitute another drug | Add a second agent from a different class (e.g., a diuretic if not selected initially) |

Inadequate Response*

Add a second or third agent, one of which should be a diuretic, if not already prescribed

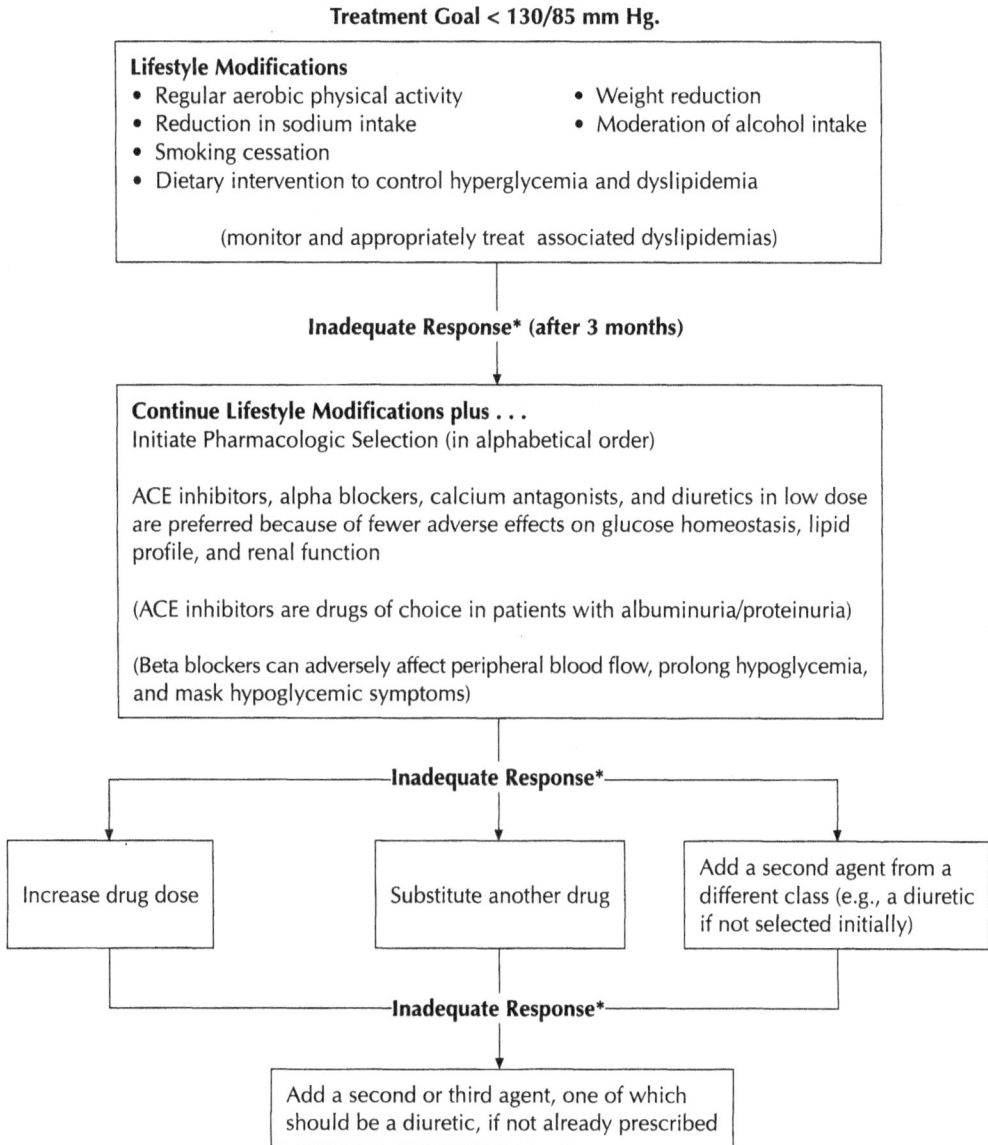

*An adequate response means goal blood pressure achieved or considerable progress made.

Figure 1. Treatment algorithm depicting a suggested approach to hypertension therapy in diabetic individuals. *Source:* Reproduced with permission from National High Blood Pressure Education Program Working Group, "National High Blood Pressure Education Program Working Group Report on Hypertension in Diabetes," *Hypertension,* Vol. 23, 145–158, © 1994, American Heart Association.

patients with NIDDM was twice as great compared to patients without diabetes.[21] Conversely, Warram and colleagues found an increase in cardiovascular mortality in 759 hypertensive diabetic patients receiving diuretic therapy.[22] This finding is supported by another study, which reported a similar outcome for hypertensive diabetics receiving diuretic therapy.[23]

These conflicting results have fostered, in part, divergent opinions on the role of diuretic and beta-blocker therapies in patients with diabetes. Regardless, many consensus statements support low-dose diuretics for the treatment of hypertension in the diabetic population.[3,13,14] Other antihypertensive therapies (e.g., ACE inhibitors, calcium channel antagonists, and alpha blockers) are currently being evaluated in ongoing trials that are designed to evaluate the impact of treatment on morbidity and mortality in hypertensive patients.

The clinical implications of insulin resistance are a possible effect on blood pressure, lipids, and obesity. Antihypertensive agents have varying effects on insulin sensitivity. In general, ACE inhibitors, alpha blockers, and calcium channel antagonists improve insulin sensitivity and lipidemia, or are lipid neutral.[24-26] Conversely, beta blockers and diuretics may worsen insulin sensitivity and the lipid profile (see Table 1).[27,28] Electrolyte imbalances may be provoked by ACE inhibitors and diuretics. Although it is unclear if these possible drug-induced changes produce clinically relevant changes in the long-term, it would seem prudent to consider these effects in each diabetic patient at the time the decision is made to initiate a specific agent to treat high blood pressure. For example, in a patient with documented hyperinsulinemia or insulin resistance, it may be prudent to select an agent that does not worsen insulin sensitivity.

Pharmacologic selection to treat blood pressure in patients with diabetes should also take into consideration the patient's concomitant disease states, medical history, and ability to pay for medications. In doing so, an antihypertensive that has a proven beneficial impact on other disease states, independent of its effect on blood pressure, may be prescribed. For example, an ACE inhibitor may be considered over other antihypertensive therapies in a patient who has diabetes and also has congestive heart failure or left ventricular hypertrophy.[29-31] Similarly, an alpha blocker may be favored if the patient suffers from benign prostatic hypertrophy. Therefore, the efficacy of the agent to control blood pressure and its effect on body chemistry should be considered in concert with its documented benefit in other disease states (see Table 2). Ultimately, drug therapy will be doomed to failure, regardless of its efficacy and beneficial effects on other disease states, if the patient cannot afford to pay for the medication.

Perhaps the most important consideration is to treat hypertension, diabetes, and dyslipidemia aggressively, as each is associated with significant morbidity and mortality.[3] Therefore, in striving to attain optimal blood pressure control, the same effort should be directed to maintain glycemic control. Intensive insulin therapy in IDDM has been reported to delay the onset and slow the progression of diabetic neuropathy, retinopathy, and nephropathy.[32] It is unknown, however, if intensive insulin therapy in NIDDM would produce similar outcomes. As insulin resistance may play more of a role in the progression and severity of diabetic complications in patients with NIDDM, insulin therapy may be withheld until oral agents have been initiated and optimized. To this end, patients with NIDDM may be prescribed oral sulfonylureas

Table 1. The impact of various classes of antihypertensive agents on body chemistry

	ACE inhibitors	Alpha blockers	Beta blockers	Calcium channel antagonists	Diuretics
Insulin sensitivity	↑	↑	↓	−↑	−↓
Electrolytes	−↑	−	−	−	↓↑
Lipidemia	−	↓	−↑	−	↑
Glycemia	−↓	−	↑	−	↑

Notes: ↑ = increase, ↓ = decrease, – = neutral.

Table 2. Treatment considerations with various disease states or conditions

Coexisting condition	ACE inhibitor	Alpha blocker	Beta blocker	Calcium channel antagonist	Diuretic
DM	++	++	–	+	+/–
Aged	+/–	+	+/–	++	++
CHF	+++	+/–	–	–	++
CAD	+	+	++	+/–	+/–
LVH	+	+/–	+	+	+/–

Notes: DM = diabetes mellitus; CHF = congestive heart failure; CAD = coronary artery disease; LVH = left ventricular hypertrophy; + = treatment benefit; – = treatment detriment; +/– = treatment neutral.

and, now, newer agents like metformin and acarbose in an attempt to control glycemia without aggravating insulin resistance.

Specific treatment measures and unique issues common to each specific class of antihypertensive drugs are delineated below with specific reference to the hypertensive diabetic population.

NONDRUG THERAPY

Nondrug treatment measures should always be employed prior to initiating drug therapy in diabetic patients with mild to moderate hypertension or in concert with drug therapy in diabetic patients with more severe hypertension.[3,14] Nondrug therapy, in general, should focus on the modification of lifestyle to include regular aerobic activity, an attempt to attain and maintain ideal body weight, cessation of smoking, and moderation of alcohol intake.[3,14] Dietary changes and physical activity can lead to improvements in glycemic, lipemic, and blood pressure control. For example, restricting sodium intake to less than 2.3 and or attaining up to a 10 lb. weight loss has been shown to lower blood pressure and improve glycemic control.[3] Daily alcohol intake should be limited to no more than 1 oz. of ethanol (equivalent to 24 oz. of beer, 8 oz. of wine, or 2 oz. of hard liquor). Patients should be encouraged to and assisted in smoking cessation. Lifestyle modifications may be tried for three months in order to control and maintain blood pressure before drug therapy is initiated.

ANTIHYPERTENSIVE THERAPY

ACE Inhibitors

ACE inhibitors decrease the progression of diabetic nephropathy independent of their blood–pressure-lowering properties.[33] In patients with IDDM and renal disease, ACE inhibitor therapy has been shown to reduce the combined endpoint of death, dialysis, or renal transplant by 50 percent.[33] These beneficial effects on the progression of diabetic nephropathy are also apparent in patients with NIDDM. In two recent, randomized, double-blind, placebo-controlled studies, ACE inhibitor therapy was associated with a decline in the loss of glomerular filtration rate (GFR), albuminuria, and maintenance of serum creatinine levels.[34,35] The retardation of declining GFR was observed for patients with mild (no more than 300 mg/24 hours) and overt (more than 300 mg/24 hours) proteinuria present at the start of the study. These findings are in accordance with a metaanalysis that reported that ACE inhibitors decrease proteinuria independent of the type of diabetes, stage of renal disease, or duration of therapy.[36] Other reasons that may predicate ACE inhibitor therapy in diabetic patients include the improvement in insulin sensitivity and the neutral effect on lipids. For these reasons, ACE inhibitors are the preferred antihypertensive agents in diabetic patients with microalbuminuria or overt diabetic nephropathy.[3,14]

The potential beneficial effects for ACE inhibitor therapy do, however, need to be considered along with several important associated adverse effects. Perhaps most important is that ACE inhibitors may worsen renal insufficiency. This is particularly important in those patients who have preexisting renal dysfunction and in those who are more dependent on the renin-angiotensin system to maintain adequate renal perfusion. For example, patients with severe congestive heart failure or renal artery disease should be monitored more frequently for an increase in serum creatinine. Likewise, ACE inhibitors may cause a dramatic and abrupt decline in renal function in patients with bilateral renal artery stenosis, a condition that is more common in patients with diabetes.[3] Caution should also be exercised when initiating therapy in patients with diabetes who are on diuretic therapy to avoid a more pronounced decline in blood pressure when these agents are prescribed together. As part of patient follow-up, serum electrolytes should be monitored to avoid hyperkalemia, which is associated with ACE inhibitor therapy.

Alpha-1 Blockers

Alpha-1 blockers are attractive antihypertensive medications for diabetic patients as they may produce a beneficial effect on lipids, improve insulin sensitivity, and possess a favorable adverse effect profile.[26,37] In addition, the longer-acting alpha-1 blockers can be administered once daily, which may lead to a better compliance rate. The main drawback associated with this class of agents is that they may provoke orthostatic hypotension. To limit this unwanted side effect, the lowest dose should be initially prescribed and the dose titrated slowly after sitting and standing blood pressures have been measured and evaluated. In addition, the first dose may be given just prior to bedtime. Unlike the central acting alpha agonists, peripheral alpha antagonists are less likely to be associated with a more pronounced or severe orthostatic hypotension in diabetics with known or suspected autonomic dysfunction.

Beta Blockers

Beta blockers should be considered for the treatment of hypertension in patients with diabetes under select conditions where there is a clear benefit (i.e., myocardial infarction or angina).[3] The reasons for limiting beta-blocker therapy to those patients who would obtain a demonstrable benefit from therapy are secondary to drug-related effects on metabolism and on the cardiovascular and nervous systems. Beta blockers without intrinsic sympathomimetic activity (ISA; e.g., atenolol and metoprolol) may aggravate lipids and decrease insulin sensitivity.[28] In addition, by blunting the sympathetic response to a hypoglycemic event, beta blockers can prolong recovery and mask symptoms the patient may rely on to signal an event. Further, beta blockers can increase claudication in patients with diabetes with peripheral vascular disease. However, these potential drug adverse effects may be outweighed in patients with diabetes following myocardial infarction, as acute and long-term beta-blocker therapy (without ISA) can improve morbidity and mortality.[38,39] Although beta blockers with ISA may have fewer of the above-mentioned adverse effects, they offer no clear advantage over other agents. There is also some evidence that when beta-blocker and diuretic therapies are combined in older adult obese patients, the risk of developing NIDDM is increased compared to controls.[40] For these reasons, beta-blocker therapy is usually reserved for those patients with diabetes for whom the benefits of therapy outweigh the risks and in select hypertensive diabetic patients for whom other antihypertensives are contraindicated, ineffective, or not tolerated.

Calcium Channel Antagonists

Calcium channel antagonists (CCAs), alone or in combination with other antihypertensive agents, are viable treatment options to control blood pressure in the diabetic population. In general, these agents are lipid neutral and do not interfere with diabetic control. CCAs, as a class, tend to be more effective with age, which make them an attractive therapy in older patients with NIDDM.[41] In addition, studies have shown that CCAs, with the exception of nifedipine, may improve diabetic nephropathy by decreasing proteinuria and microalbuminuria.[42] However, not all studies are in agreement with this finding, and it is unknown if this beneficial effect is maintained with continued long-term therapy.[42] It has also been proposed that an additive effect may be produced by combining a CCA with an ACE inhibitor in patients with diabetic nephropathy.[43] Clearly, more well-controlled studies are needed to clarify the impact of specific CCAs on diabetic renal disease and to determine if combination therapy with an ACE inhibitor produces a synergistic effect.

Orthostatic hypotension, constipation, and peripheral edema are the main side effects associated with CCAs. Initiating therapy at the lowest possible dose and titrating slowly may be the best means of curtailing these unwanted side effects. Also, extra caution should be exercised to avoid orthostatic hypotension in diabetics with known or suspected neuropathy. As highlighted recently in the literature, short-acting agents (e.g., nifedipine) should be avoided in general for the chronic treatment of hypertension secondary to a possible increase in the risk of myocardial infarction.[44,45]

DIURETICS

Thiazide diuretics have been shown to provoke adverse effects on lipid metabolism, blood glucose, and blood chemistry (e.g., potassium, magnesium, and urea).[13] However, when prescribed in low dose (25 mg or less a day of hydrochlorothiazide), these unwanted side effects may not be as pronounced and may be of little clinical importance.[3] Of note, loop diuretics have not been shown to have these effects and are preferred over thiazides when a patient's renal function worsens (serum creatinine greater than 2.5 mg/dL).[19] As patients with diabetes can be described as having an expanded plasma volume, diuretic therapy may be a necessary and effective therapy to control blood pressure in this population.[46] Further, combination therapy with an ACE inhibitor can produce a synergistic effect in lowering blood pressure and therefore can be considered for patients with diabetes who require more than one antihypertensive agent to control blood pressure.[47]

● ● ●

Hypertension in patients with diabetes should be treated early and aggressively. Pharmacologic and nondrug therapies combined with lifestyle modifications are important measures to achieve optimal treatment outcomes. Antihypertensive drugs, including ACE inhibitors, alpha blockers, CCAs, and low-dose diuretics, should be initiated if needed to attain and maintain optimal blood pressure control. Prior to initiating antihypertensive therapy, consideration and careful evaluation of drug-related effects on morbidity and mortality, possible effects on body chemistry, and the impact of therapy on concomitant disease states should be made. As a result, the best antihypertensive agent or combination of agents can be delineated for each patient. These measures to control hypertension should mirror efforts to optimize glycemic and lipemic control in each patient with diabetes.

REFERENCES

1. American Diabetes Association, *Diabetes 1993 Vital Statistics* (Alexandria, VA: 1993).
2. P.M. Dodson, "Epidemiology and Pathogenesis of Hypertension in Diabetes," in *Hypertension and Diabetes,* eds. A.H. Barnett and P.M. Dodson (London: Science Press, 1990).
3. The National High Blood Pressure Education Program Working Group, "National High Blood Pressure Education Program Working Group Report on Hypertension in Diabetes," *Hypertension* 23 (1994): 145–158.
4. M. Epstein, and J.R. Sowers, "Diabetes Mellitus and Hypertension," *Hypertension* 19 (1992): 403–418.
5. J.M. Flack, and J.R. Sowers, "Epidemiologic and Clinical Aspects of Insulin Resistance and Hyperinsulinemia."

American Journal of Medicine 91, suppl. 1A (1991): 11S–21S.

6. J.S. Skyler et al., "Hypertension in Patients with Diabetes Mellitus," *American Journal of Hypertension* 8 (1995): 100S–105S.

7. A.R. Christlieb et al., "Vascular Reactivity to Angiotensin II and to Noradrenaline in Diabetic Subjects," *Diabetes* 25 (1976): 268–274.

8. R.A. De Fronzo, "The Effect of Insulin on Renal Sodium Metabolism," *Diabetologia* 21 (1981): 165–171.

9. P. Weidmann et al., "Pressor Factors and Responsiveness in Hypertension Accompanying Diabetes Mellitus," *Hypertension* 7, suppl. 2 (1985): 43–48.

10. P.M. Bell, "Clinical Significance of Insulin Resistance," *Diabetic Medicine* 13 (1996): 504–509.

11. R.E. Gilbert et al., "Diabetes and Hypertension. Australian Diabetes Society Position Statement," *The Medical Journal of Australia* 163 (1995): 372–375.

12. K.G. Dawson et al., "Report of the Canadian Hypertension Society Consensus Conference: 5. Hypertension and Diabetes," *Canadian Medical Association Journal* 149 (1993): 821–826.

13. American Diabetes Association, "Treatment of Hypertension in Diabetes," *Diabetes Care* 16 (1993): 1,394–1,401.

14. J.R. Sowers, and M. Epstein, "Diabetes Mellitus and Associated Hypertension, Vascular Disease, and Nephropathy: An Update," *Hypertension* 26, part 1 (1995): 869–879.

15. S. MacMahon et al., "Blood Pressure, Stroke, and Coronary Heart Disease. Part 1: Prolonged Differences in Blood Pressure: Prospective Observational Studies Corrected for the Regression Dilution Bias," *Lancet* 335 (1990): 765–774.

16. Medical Research Council Working Party, "Medical Research Council Trial of Treatment of Hypertension in Older Adults: Principal Results," *British Medical Journal* 304 (1992): 405–412.

17. B. Dahlof et al., "Morbidity and Mortality in the Swedish Trial in Old Patients with Hypertension (STOP-Hypertension)," *Lancet* 338 (1991): 1,281–1,285.

18. R. Collins et al., "Blood Pressure, Stroke, and Coronary Heart Disease. Part 2: Short-term Reductions in Blood Pressure: Overview of Randomized Drug Trials in their Epidemiological Context," *Lancet* 335 (1990): 827–838.

19. Joint National Committee, "The Fifth Report of the Joint National Committee on Detection, Evaluation, and Treatment of High Blood Pressure," *Archives of Internal Medicine* 153 (1993): 154–183.

20. SHEP Cooperative Research Group, "Prevention of Stroke by Antihypertensive Drug Treatment in Older Persons with Isolated Systolic Hypertension: Final Results of the Systolic Hypertension in the Elderly Program (SHEP)," *JAMA* 265 (1991): 3,255–3,264.

21. J.D. Curb et al., "Effect of Diuretic-based Antihypertensive Treatment on Cardiovascular Disease in Older Diabetic Patients with Isolated Systolic Hypertension," *JAMA* 276 (1996): 1,886–1,892.

22. J.H. Warram et al., "Excess Mortality Associated with Diuretic Therapy in Diabetes Mellitus," *Archives of Internal Medicine* 151 (1991): 1,350–1,356.

23. R. Klein et al., "Relation of Ocular and Systemic Factors to Survival in Diabetes," *Archives of Internal Medicine* 149 (1989): 266–272.

24. T. Pollare et al., "A Comparison of the Effects of Hydrochlorothiazide and Captopril on Glucose and Lipid Metabolism in Patients with Hypertension," *New England Journal of Medicine* 321 (1989): 868–873.

25. W.H.H. Sheu et al., "Comparison of the Effects of Atenolol and Nifedipine on Glucose, Insulin, and Lipid Metabolism in Patients with Hypertension," *American Journal of Hypertension* 4 (1991): 199–205.

26. A. Lehtonen, "Doxazosin Effects on Insulin and Glucose in Hypertensive Patients. The Finnish Multicenter Study Group," *American Heart Journal* 121 (1991): 1,307–1,311.

27. H.O. Lithell, "Effect of Antihypertensive Drugs on Insulin, Glucose, and Lipid Metabolism," *Diabetes Care* 14 (1991): 203–209.

28. T. Pollare et al., "Sensitivity to Insulin During Treatment with Atenolol and Metoprolol: A Randomized, Double Blind Study of Effects on Carbohydrate and Lipoprotein Metabolism in Hypertensive Patients," *British Medical Journal* 298 (1989): 1,152–1,157.

29. SOLVD Investigators, "Effect of Enalapril on Survival in Patients with Reduced Left Ventricular Ejection Fractions and Congestive Heart Failure," *New England Journal of Medicine* 325 (1991): 293–302.

30. SOLVD Investigators, "Effect of Enalapril on Mortality and the Development of Heart Failure in Asymptomatic Patients with Reduced Left-ventricular Ejection Fractions," *New England Journal of Medicine* 327 (1992): 685–691.

31. F.G. Dunn et al., "Enalapril Improves Systemic and Renal Hemodynamics and Allows Regression of Left Ventricular Mass in Essential Hypertension," *American Journal of Cardiology* 53 (1984): 105–108.

32. The Diabetes Control and Complications Trial Research Group, "The Effect of Intensive Treatment of Diabetes on the Development and Progression of Long Term Complications in Insulin Dependent Diabetes Mellitus," *New England Journal of Medicine* 329 (1993): 977–986.

33. E.J. Lewis et al. for the Collaborative Study Group, "The Effect of Angiotensin-converting Enzyme Inhibition on Diabetic Nephropathy," *New England Journal of Medicine* 329 (1993): 1,456–1,462.

34. H.E. Lebovitz et al., "Renal Protective Effects of Enalapril in Hypertensive NIDDM: Role of Baseline Albuminuria," *Kidney International* 45 (1994): S150–S155.

35. M. Ravid et al., "Long-term Stabilizing Effect of Angiotensin-converting Enzyme Inhibition on Plasma Creatinine and on Proteinuria in Normotensive Type II Diabetic Patients," *Annals of Internal Medicine* 118 (1993): 577–581.

36. B.L. Kasiske et al., "Effect of Antihypertensive Therapy on the Kidney in Patients with Diabetes: A Meta-regression Analysis," *Annals of Internal Medicine* 118 (1993): 129–138.

37. R.R. Luther et al., "The Effects of Terazosin and Methylchlorothiazide on Blood Pressure and Serum Lipids," *American Heart Journal* 117 (1989): 842–847.

38. ISIS-1 (First International Study of Infarct Survival) Collaborative Group, "Randomized Trial of Intravenous Atenolol Among 16,027 Cases of Suspected Acute Myocardial Infarction: ISIS-1," *Lancet* 12 (1986): 57–66.

39. G. Olsson et al., "Long-term Treatment with Metoprolol after Acute MI: Effect on 3 Year Mortality and Morbidity," *Journal of the American College of Cardiology* 5 (1985): 1,428–1,437.

40. L. Mykkanen et al., "Increased Risk of Non-insulin Dependent Diabetes in Elderly Hypertensive Subjects," *Journal of Hypertension* 12 (1994): 1,425–1,432.

41. W. Zing et al., "Calcium Antagonists in Elderly and Black Hypertensive Patients," *Archives of Internal Medicine* 151 (1991): 2,154–2,162.

42. D.D. Hoelscher et al., "Hypertension in Diabetic Patients: An Update of Interventional Studies to Preserve Renal Function," *Journal of Clinical Pharmacology* 35 (1995): 73–80.

43. G.L. Bakris et al., "Treatment of Arterial Hypertension in Diabetic Humans: Importance of Therapeutic Selection," *Kidney International* 41 (1992): 912–919.

44. B.M. Psaty et al. "The Risk of Myocardial Infarction Associated with Antihypertensive Drug Therapies," *JAMA* 274 (1995): 620–625.

45. B.G. Phillips et al., "Calcium-channel Blockers and Risk of Myocardial Infarction: More Hype than Harm," *American Journal of Health System Pharmacy* 52 (1995): 1,460–1,462.

46. G.W. Edelson, and J.R. Sowers, "Treatment of Hypertension in Selected Patient Groups: An Emphasis on Diabetes Mellitus and Hypertension," *The Endocrinologist* 4 (1995): 205–210.

47. B. Dahlof et al., "Controlled Trial or Enalapril and Hydrochlorothiazide in 200 Hypertensive Patients," *American Journal of Hypertension* 1 (1988): 38–41.

CHAPTER 11

Issues in Treating the
Geriatric Patient with Diabetes

Gordon A. Ireland, PharmD

Diabetes, a disease commonly seen in the young, is more frequently seen in the geriatric age group (older than 65 years of age). This frequency has been estimated at 30 to 50 percent, although because of underdiagnosis, reported cases have approximately a 20 percent occurrence, the majority of which is Type II or non–insulin-dependent diabetes (NIDDM). Although the presentation in older adults is similar to that in younger patients, there are considerations for both evaluation and therapy that are unique to the geriatric patient. Key words: *acarbose, biguanide, geriatric, insulin, NIDDM, sulfonylurea*

Type II or non–insulin-dependent diabetes mellitus (NIDDM) is commonly seen in the geriatric age group (older than 65 years of age). Twenty percent of this population has been diagnosed with NIDDM, although, due to underdiagnosis, the frequency has been estimated at 30 to 50 percent.[1] More than half of these cases are in females, and those who have undergone multiple childbirths have a greater statistical chance of developing diabetes. The hyperglycemia associated with NIDDM occurs because of a combination of factors: impaired glucose uptake into skeletal muscle cells due to insulin resistance; increased hepatic glucose production; and initially, impaired second phase pancreatic insulin secretion, followed, later in the course of the disease, by impaired first phase secretion. If left untreated, NIDDM is associated with the development of retinopathy, nephropathy, neuropathy, and atherosclerotic disease, which cause a 10 percent decrease in the 10-year survival rate of geriatric patients.[2] The evaluation and treatment of NIDDM in the older patient must consider factors that may differ from those seen in younger patients, including risk

factors, complications, symptoms, goals of therapy, and special considerations when choosing a therapeutic modality.

RISK FACTORS

The risk factors for NIDDM include physiological changes due to the aging process, a sedentary lifestyle, complications of other diseases, hereditary factors, female gender, parity, and obesity. (See box, "Risk Factors for NIDDM.") The physiological changes that occur during the aging process are numerous, some of which increase the development of NIDDM, while others affect the complications of the disease and the choice of treatment. Aging causes a decrease in insulin production by the pancreas and a decrease both in the number of insulin receptors and in the sensitivity of these receptors to the effect of insulin, which results in an inability to control the blood glucose level. Although these changes generally occur in all individuals, they are of greater significance in individuals with a family history of NIDDM. This decrease in glucose control is exacerbated by obesity, which

---

Risk Factors For NIDDM

- physiological changes
- lifestyle changes
- complications of other diseases
- heredity
- female gender
- number of childbirths
- obesity

---

may be a result of diets higher in carbohydrates and fat, and a more sedentary lifestyle, causing an even greater insulin requirement.[3] Neurological changes of aging are associated with decreasing rate and amplitude of the nervous signals leading to compromised sensory input, decreased coordination, increased falls, and a slowing of mental function. These changes may become significantly worse in patients with NIDDM. Decreased thirst mechanism makes it more difficult to maintain adequate hydration when higher glucose levels produce an osmotic diuresis. Decreased visual acuity may compromise the patient's ability to monitor blood glucose levels and measure insulin doses, if use of insulin becomes necessary. The age-related slowing of renal glomerular filtration rate (GFR) and decreasing liver function may contraindicate the use of certain therapeutic modalities. The interaction of other diseases, such as dementia, depression, chronic renal failure, arthritis, and malnutrition, may make the evaluation and management of NIDDM much more difficult.[3]

COMPLICATIONS OF NIDDM

The long-term complications of NIDDM, although common to both types of diabetes, seem to occur more rapidly and more severely in the geriatric patient, possibly because the diagnosis is made at a later time in the course of the disease or the complications are superimposed on similar changes occurring due to the aging process.[3] (See box, "Complications of NIDDM.") Chronic complications include vascular, neurological, metabolic, visual, and immunological.

Acute complications that occur when blood glucose levels rise are slowing of mental function, blurring of vision, difficulty differentiating colors, polyuria, and polydypsia.

Vascular

Diabetes-induced vascular diseases are classified as either macrovascular (large vessel) or microvascular (small vessel) disease. These diseases are due to atherosclerotic changes that occur within the vessels and decreased blood flow to the affected areas. Macrovascular disease is accelerated by diabetes.[4] NIDDM patients are more likely to have coronary artery disease with resultant angina and myocardial infarction; cerebrovascular disease producing decreased mental function and ischemic strokes; and peripheral vascular disease resulting in a decreased ability to combat local infections leading to possible gangrene with an accompanying amputation of toes, feet, or even legs. Macrovascular changes have also been implicated in sexual dysfunctions. In females, vaginal dryness is associated with painful intercourse and increased vaginal infections, and in males, erectile dysfunction, also caused by neurological complications, is the primary problem. Retinal abnormalities associated with steadily deteriorating visual acuity and renal disease producing decreased kidney function and protein loss are a result of the microvascular changes and neuropathies of NIDDM.[5]

Neurological

Neurological complications of NIDDM include both central and peripheral effects. The

---

Complications of NIDDM

- macrovascular disease
- microvascular disease
- neurological
- metabolic
- visual
- immunological

---

central nervous system slowing causes cognitive impairment evidenced by a slowing of the thought process and memory retrieval.[6] This effect may be exacerbated by the diabetic vascular changes and the aging process.[7] Depression is also more common in diabetic older adults than the same age group without diabetes.[8] Peripheral neuropathy produces significantly decreased sensory input leading to the patient's inability to feel pain. This decreased sensation allows foot cuts to go undetected and, in conjunction with peripheral vascular disease, may eventually lead to amputation of the extremity. Two thirds of amputations occur in patients over the age of 65, and two thirds of these are in individuals with diabetes.[9] While pain sensation transmission is decreased in peripheral neuropathic neurons, the pain sensation of peripheral neuropathy is increased in patients with diabetes. One study showed that patients with diabetes complain of pain more frequently than nondiabetic controls exhibiting both an earlier stimulus detection and a decreased pain tolerance.[10] The same study found similar results when blood glucose levels were increased in nondiabetic subjects.

Metabolic

Metabolic abnormalities include hyperlipidemia and atherosclerosis in NIDDM. These abnormalities lead to coronary artery disease and peripheral vascular disease.

Visual

Diabetic retinopathy, which can lead to decreased visual acuity and color blindness, increases with age from 10 percent at age 55 to about 30 percent at age 80. Cataracts and glaucoma also occur with greater frequency in patients with diabetes than in similarly aged nondiabetic patients.[11] The color blindness produces a difficulty in differentiating shades of color. This may cause the misinterpretation of color-mediated tests in diabetes monitoring. Patients may also have blurring of vision intermittently when glucose levels are high because of increased glucose concentrations in the humors of

the eye. Although the blurring can be corrected as the blood glucose levels are brought back to normal, it may have serious consequences when it occurs in patients who already have age-related visual changes.

Immunological

Immunological deficiency associated with NIDDM in older patients puts them at risk for the occurrence of a greater number of infections.[11] These infections include pulmonary, genitourinary tract, cuts, and diabetic foot ulcers, which are more difficult to treat and take longer to heal.

SYMPTOMS

The symptoms of diabetes in the older adult patient are similar to those in the young (i.e., polyuria, polydypsia, polyphagia, weakness, lethargy, and blurred vision). However, some differences do exist. Older patients frequently have nocturia as a result of benign prostatic hypertrophy (BPH), smaller bladder size, and other diseases due to the aging process or the more frequent use of diuretics. These other causes of nocturia must be distinguished from hyperglycemia. Polydypsia may not be obvious since decreased thirst sensitivity occurs with advancing age. Increased appetite may also not be noticeable since satiety occurs more readily in the geriatric patient. Weakness, lethargy, and blurred vision may appear as a result of aging, concurrent diseases, and/or medications consumed. It is, therefore, important to consider these differences when evaluating the geriatric patient.

GOALS OF THERAPY

The primary goal for therapy of the geriatric patient with NIDDM is to maintain fasting blood glucose (FBG) levels below 140 mg/dL, all random blood glucose (RBG) levels below 200 mg/dL, and a hemoglobin A$_{1c}$ (HbA$_{1c}$) below 8 percent.[12] Achieving this goal will usually prevent the symptoms of hyperglycemia. Although the long-term advantage of treating asymptomatic hyperglycemia in the "old old" (older than 80 years of age) has not been documented, glycemic control does prevent acute symptoms.[12] Tighter control may be necessary to prevent long-term complications (i.e., FBG less than 115 mg/dL and RBG less than 180 mg/dL, and HbA$_{1c}$ less than 7 percent).[12] If the primary goal is accomplished, other goals, such as decreased incidence of symptoms, prevention of hyperosmolar coma, and prevention of ketoacidotic or lactic acidotic hyperglycemic coma will be achieved. The microvascular long-term complications may be prevented by glycemic control, but data do not support the prevention of macrovascular complications in Type II diabetes.[13] (See box, "Goals of Therapy.") Above all, the goal should be to improve the quality of life of the patient. The therapy or the monitoring procedure should not decrease the quality of life.

SPECIAL CONSIDERATIONS IN THERAPY

There are many age-related considerations that must be addressed when treating diabetes in the older adult patient, such as altered vision, dietary changes, musculoskeletal abnormalities, cognitive function impairment, decreased renal function, and other medications.

Altered Vision

Altered vision may make it more difficult, if not impossible, to perform self-monitoring procedures and drawing insulin into the syringe. It is imperative to watch older patients performing these functions to ensure their capability. This observing may be performed by any trained health

---

Goals of Therapy

- Control blood glucose levels.
- Decrease the incidence of symptoms.
- Prevent, reduce, or improve complications.
- Improve quality of life.

---

professional and should not be limited to physicians or nurses. Pharmacists are ideally positioned to perform this role in hospitals, in home care, and especially in retail pharmacies when patients come to have their prescriptions filled. If patients are unable, family members can be trained or arrangements made for a visiting health professional to draw up the insulin and/or perform the monitoring tasks. Again, pharmacists could supply prefilled syringes and arrange the monitoring.

Dietary Changes

Decreased appetite may make it difficult for patients to maintain a diabetic diet and, if they are taking insulin or an oral hypoglycemic agent, may produce periods of hypoglycemia. A diary should be maintained for recording daily dietary intake, exercise involvement, blood glucose levels, and medication doses, if needed. The age-related decreased thirst sensitivity may result in dehydration, causing orthostatic hypotension and the possibility of sustaining an injury from a fall.

Musculoskeletal Abnormalities

Tremors and arthritis may also compromise patients' ability to take care of their therapy and monitoring. Poor dexterity secondary to decreased joint mobility, muscle tremor, muscle weakness, and decreased coordination make it difficult to perform the mechanics of performing monitoring tests and, if necessary, drawing up insulin. As with the visual abnormalities, provision must be made to perform these functions for the patient.

Cognitive Function Problems

Impaired cognitive function and memory dysfunction may make it difficult for the patient to remember instructions and perform monitoring and therapeutic tasks. If the patient is unable to repeat instructions and perform monitoring and therapeutic activities, family members should be trained or arrangements made for a visiting health professional to draw up and administer the insulin and/or perform the monitoring tasks.

Decreased Renal Function

The decreased renal function associated with the aging process must be considered when choosing the therapeutic modality in the older adult diabetic patient. Since serum creatinine measurements in geriatric patients are usually within normal range despite a 30 to 50 percent decrease in GFR,[14] a creatinine clearance should be measured or calculated to better determine kidney function prior to starting therapy.

Other Medications

Many older patients are taking other medications that may cause an increase in blood glucose levels or may interact with the diabetes therapy (e.g., diuretics, corticosteroids, beta blockers). These problems may be avoided by performing a thorough medication history prior to the initiation of any therapy. The same caution may be applied to the interaction between diabetes and other disease states since older individuals tend to have multiple maladies (e.g., decreased renal function, decreased neurological function, and Parkinson's disease).

Other Considerations

Other considerations include decreased physical activity, economics of therapy, medication interactions, and disease interactions. Decreased physical activity can lead to a lower requirement of glucose intake but an increased need for insulin. This combination is extremely difficult to control in a sedentary geriatric patient, who produces less insulin, and it may exacerbate the occurrence of NIDDM. Since many geriatric patients are living on low fixed incomes, the cost of the proposed therapy and monitoring should be carefully considered. Some choices of therapy and monitoring are less expensive than others. The least costly medication that will fit the patient's needs should be chosen, and monitoring tests should be done as infrequently as possible. For example, in a controlled patient, home glucose monitoring could be done once every other day or even less frequently, if deemed adequate. Performing the test at a different time each test day will eventually produce data to evaluate the patient's glycemic control over the whole day without the cost and trauma of multiple tests per day.

THERAPY

Diabetes therapy in older adults requires a team approach in order to address all the issues involved. The input of physicians, nurses, pharmacists, dietitians, physical therapists, social workers, family, and friends must all be considered to maximize the patient's therapy for the attainment of the best possible outcome. The therapy also should have a multilayered approach. (See box, "Therapeutic Options.")

Nonpharmacological Therapy

The nonpharmacological aspects of therapy in the older adult diabetic patient with NIDDM are possibly more important to the achievement of the desired outcome than the medications. It is extremely important that a good base be established on which to apply the needed medication therapy. The components to the base are diet, exercise, lifestyle changes, and education.

Diet

Dietary therapy should be aimed at weight stabilization. If the patient is overweight, weight reduction will aid in the control of the hyperglycemia. NIDDM patients who are overweight and being treated with oral hypoglycemic agents have been able to discontinue the medications after weight reduction. Patients who are underweight due to decreased nutritional intake need

---

Therapeutic Options

- diet
- exercise
- behavioral modification
- sulfonylureas
- metformin
- acarbose
- insulin

to increase their body weight to a more ideal amount. Diets incorporating nutritional foods governed by the calorie intake to maintain the patient's ideal body weight, have been successful in producing weight stabilization and aiding in glucose control.[15] The dietary program should also be low in fat since hyperlipidemia and atherosclerosis are more prevalent in patients with diabetes. Dietary therapy alone is not sufficient but must be used in conjunction with exercise and behavioral changes.

Exercise

A planned program of exercise developed specifically for each individual patient is the second leg of this therapeutic base. Exercise has multiple benefits for the patient. It improves the body's ability to move glucose into skeletal muscle cells with a decreased need for insulin, burns calories, improves tissue oxygenation, improves muscle strength, improves coordination, and ultimately improves the patient's quality of life.[16] Although any amount of exercise is beneficial, it maybe difficult to achieve the necessary amount in the older patient due to underlying conditions (e.g., multiple disease states, arthritis, and osteoporosis).

Lifestyle

Lifestyle changes involve not only changing diet and starting an exercise program but also stopping smoking, drinking alcoholic beverages sparingly, adopting a less sedentary lifestyle, and avoiding stress-producing situations. It may be very difficult, however, to make some changes in the lifestyle of a 90-year-old patient. If smoking is this person's only "pleasure in life," it will be almost impossible, and maybe unnecessary, to stop that behavior. Each lifestyle change must be analyzed not only on its impact on disease therapy but also on how it will affect the patient's quality of life.

Education

If diet, exercise, and behavioral modification are the legs for the therapy base, education is necessary to stabilize them. Diabetes control is more likely to occur in patients who are well educated

not only about their disease and the end results of the disease but also about all aspects of nonpharmacological and, if necessary, pharmacological therapy and monitoring procedures. (See box, "Therapeutic Options.") The patient must buy into the total package in order for the treatment to be successful. It is also very important to involve the patient's family in this process because they will be the patient's daily support and compliance advocates.

Pharmacological Therapy

Pharmacological therapy for NIDDM in the older adult patient should only be started in severe hyperglycemia or after nonpharmacological modalities have been unsuccessful in controlling the blood glucose levels. (See box, "Hypoglycemic Agents.")

Sulfonylureas

Sulfonylureas are usually the first choice of second generation medication therapy since they produce a more predictable hypoglycemic response than the first generation.[17] Chlorpropamide is the only sulfonylurea that should not be used in the geriatric patient because it has a very long half-life (t1/2) and multiple adverse reac-

---

Hypoglycemic Agents

1. Sulfonylureas
   - first generation
     - tolazamide (Tolinase)
     - tolbutamide (Orinase)
     - acetohexamide (Dymelor)
     - chlorpropamide (Diabinese)
   - second generation
     - glyburide (Micronase, Diabeta)
     - glipizide (Glucotrol, Glucotrol XL)
     - glimepiride (Amaryl)
2. Biguanide
   - metformin (Glucophage)
3. Alpha-glucosidase inhibitor
   - acarbose (Precose)
4. Insulin

tions.[18] The second generation sulfonylureas have equivalent hypoglycemic effects and differ primarily in their duration of hypoglycemic activity. In older adult patients glipizide usually needs to be administered twice a day, glyburide, is usually effective when given once daily due to a slightly longer half-life,[19] while glimepiride should only be given once daily. The once-daily dosing of glyburide and glimepiride should produce a better compliance to therapy. Doses in older adult patients should always be started at the lowest dose and titrated upward based on the patient's response. The two primary concerns with sulfonylureas are weight gain and hypoglycemia, both of which can usually be kept to a minimum by good patient education and follow-up.[20]

Biguanide

Metformin is usually prescribed as a second choice in older adult patients with NIDDM and may be added to or substituted for the sulfonylurea.[21] The reason for this placement is the potential for lactic acidosis, which occurs in patients with decreased renal function (creatinine less than 60 ml/min.), a common finding in the geriatric patient. Metformin should be used with caution in patients with decreased GFR.[22] Metformin also needs to be discontinued for any situation in which the patient has the potential of experiencing low blood pressure to the point of compromising renal function. It should not be administered to persons with cardiac failure, liver disease, and chronic acidosis.[23] The possible advantages of metformin over sulfonylureas are no weight gain, more likely weight loss, and less potential for hypoglycemic episodes.

Alpha-glucosidase Inhibitor

Acarbose, due to its side effect profile, multiple daily dosing regimen, and lower efficacy, should not be used as initial therapy in the geriatric patient with diabetes but may be useful as an addition to a sulfonylurea, especially if the lack of control is due to postprandial hyperglycemia.[24] Acarbose is not recommended for use in patients with cirrhosis or with renal impairment (serum creatinine greater than 2.0 mg/dL). Great caution must be used in the geriatric patient until creatinine clearance cautionary data are available, since normal serum creatinine levels may be obtained despite 50 to 60 percent renal function.

Insulin

Insulin should be used to treat older adult patients with NIDDM only after a trial of oral therapy has failed. Insulin may cause weight gain in NIDDM patients, which leads to the need for more insulin, causing more weight gain, resulting in steadily increasing doses of insulin in response to the patient's gain in weight. If used correctly, however, insulin is of benefit both in controlling hyperglycemia and preventing some end organ damage.[25] Insulin self-administration by the geriatric diabetic patient may be compromised by decreased visual acuity, tremor, arthritis, and decreased cognitive function.

NIDDM treatment in the geriatric patient should be initiated with maximum nonpharmacological interventions followed by a sulfonylurea (glyburide or glipizide). If this regimen fails, the addition of metformin or acarbose, if they are not contraindicated, may improve glucemic control. Insulin therapy should be reserved until a program of nonpharmacological combined with oral hypoglycemic agents has been unsuccessful.

MONITORING

Disease and therapy monitoring in the older adult diabetic patient should be accomplished through a combination of laboratory and self-monitoring with a goal of achieving an FBG of less than 140 mg/dL, an RBG of less than 200 mg/dL, and a glycosylated hemoglobin of less than 8 percent. Self-monitoring by the geriatric with diabetes may be compromised by decreased visual acuity, tremor, arthritis, and decreased cognitive function.

• • •

In conclusion, diabetes control in older persons may decrease complications and should improve quality of life, but special attention needs to be given to the potential problems associated with this patient group. Patients should be observed administering medications and performing self-monitoring tests by a health care professional to ensure their capability. If incapable, family, friends, or home care professionals may be needed to administer the medications and perform the

testing. Patients should also be encouraged to keep a detailed diary of glucose values, times tested, medication administration, dietary intake, exercise participation, and any signs or symptoms of hyper- or hypoglycemia. A well-educated and supported geriatric patient is a necessity if NIDDM therapy is to be successful.

REFERENCES

1. M.I. Harris et al., "Prevalence of Diabetes and Impaired Glucose Tolerance and Plasma Glucose Levels in US Population, Ages 24–74 Years," *Diabetes* 36 (1987): 523.

2. B.D. Naliboff, and M. Rosenthal, *Effects of Age on Complications in Adult-Onset Diabetes,* 37 (1989): 383–843.

3. M.J. Rosenthal et al., "Diabetes in the Elderly," *Journal of the American Geriatric Society* 35 (1987): 435–447.

4. R.P. Donahue, and T.J. Orchard, "Diabetes Mellitus and Macrovascular Complications: An Epidemiological Perspective," *Diabetes Care* 15 (1992): 1,141–1,155.

5. P. Reichard et al., "The Effect of Long-Term Intensified Treatment on the Development of Microvascular Complications of Diabetes Mellitus," *New England Journal of Medicine* 329 (1993): 304–309.

6. G.M. Reaven et al., "Relationship between Hyperglycemia and Cognitive Function in Older NIDDM Patients," *Diabetes Care* 13 (1990): 16–21.

7. R.C. Uren et al., "The Mental Efficiency of the Elderly Person with Type II Diabetes Mellitus," *Journal of the American Geriatric Society* 38 (1990): 505–510.

8. L.J. Fitten, "ULA Geriatric Grand Rounds: Depression." *Journal of the American Geriatric Society* 37 (1989): 459–472.

9. J.E. Morley et al., "Diabetes in Elderly Patients: Is it Different?" *American Journal of Medicine* 83 (1987): 533–544.

10. J.E. Morley et al., "Why Is Diabetic Peripheral Neuropathy Painful? The Effect of Glucose on Pain Perception in Humans," *American Journal of Medicine* 77 (1984): 79–83.

11. L.G. Lipson, "Diabetes in the Elderly: Diagnosis, Pathogenesis, and Therapy," *American Journal of Medicine* 80, suppl. 5A (1986): 10–21.

12. D. Nathan et al., "Glycemic Control in Diabetes Mellitus: Have Changes in Therapy Made a Difference?" *American Journal of Medicine* 100, no. 2 (1996): 157–163.

13. G. Meneilly, "The Effect of Improved Glycemic Control on Cognitive Functions in the Elderly Patient with Diabetes," *Journal of Gerontology* 48 (1993): M117–M121.

14. R.D. Lindeman, "Changes in Renal Function with Aging: Implications for Treatment," *Drugs and Aging* 2 (1992): 423–431.

15. F.E. Kaiser, and M.J. Rosenthal, "Nutrition and Diabetes Mellitus in the Elderly," in *Geriatric Nutrition,* ed. J.E. Morley (New York: Raven Press, 1990).

16. E.T. Skarfors et al., "Physical Training as Treatment for Type II (Non-insulin Dependent) Diabetes in Elderly Men. A Feasibility Study Over 2 Years," *Diabetologia* 30 (1987): 930–933.

17. N. Melander et al., "Sulfonylureas. Why, Which, and How?" *Diabetes Care* (1990): 18–25.

18. J.A. Tayler "Pharmacokinetics and Biotransformation of Chlorpropamide in Man," *Clinical Pharmacology and Therapeutics* 13 (1972): 710–718.

19. L.A. Jaber et al., "An Evaluation of the Therapeutic Effects and Dosage Equivalence of Glyburide and Glipizide," *Journal of Clinical Pharmacology* 30 (1990): 181–188.

20. M. Stepka et al., "Hypoglycemia: A Major Problem in the Management of Diabetes in the Elderly," *Aging* 5 (1993): 117–121.

21. C. Bailey, "Biguanides and NIDDM," *Diabetes Care* 15 (1992): 755–772.

22. R. DeFronzo, and A. Goodman, "Multicenter Metformin Study Group. Efficacy of Metformin in Patients with Non-insulin Diabetes Mellitus," *New England Journal of Medicine* 339 (1995): 541–549.

23. W.R. Melchior, and L.A. Jaber, "An Antihyperglycemic Agent for Treatment of Type II Diabetes," *Annals of Pharmacotherapy* 30 (1996): 158–163.

24. J. Chiasson et al., "The Efficacy of Acarbose in the Treatment of Patients with Non-insulin Dependent Diabetes Mellitus," *Annals of Internal Medicine* 121 (1994): 928–935.

25. S.V. Edelman et al., "Intensive Insulin Therapy for Patients with Type II Diabetes," *Current Opinion in Endocrinology and Diabetes* 2 (1995): 333–340.

CHAPTER 12

Systematic Approach to the Management of the Type II Diabetic Patient: Case Presentation

Lenore T. Coleman, PharmD, CDE, FASHP

Recently there has been a trend toward more aggressive management of people with diabetes. This stems from the conclusive clinical data that substantiate the benefit of tight glycemic control. It is clear that achieving near normoglycemia in people with diabetes will prevent and slow the progression of the microvascular complications and reduce the risk of the macrovascular complications. Clinicians now have multiple agents with differing mechanisms and sites of action allowing them to individualize the medication regimen and move toward normalizing the blood glucose levels. The following case is representative of a typical patient with Type II diabetes. This patient presents with multiple disease states and various treatment issues that must be addressed. An indepth evaluation of the patient case is presented along with recommendations for drug therapy modifications. Key words: *acarbose, antidiabetic agents, case management, Type II diabetes*

Diabetes is a significant chronic disease affecting people of all age groups and ethnicities. It has become a major clinical and public health problem in the United States. According to the most recent statistics published by the American Diabetes Association and National Institutes of Health, an estimated 16 million Americans have Type I or Type II diabetes. There are approximately 800,000 people with insulin-dependent diabetes (Type I) and approximately seven million with non–insulin-dependent diabetes (Type II).[1] Eight million of these patients have been formally diagnosed and know that they have the disease; the other eight million are undiagnosed.[1–3] Interestingly, a survey of people with diabetes indicates that 50 percent of cases are detected "by chance."[1]

Diabetes is the sixth leading cause of death from disease in the United States and accounts for 5 to 6 percent of hospital admissions. It is estimated that 169,000 deaths from diabetes occurred in 1992.[2] This figure is probably an underestimate due to inaccurate recording of "cause of death." Another 20 million Americans have impaired glucose tolerance (IGT), a condition that is diagnosed when the fasting plasma glucose is less than 140 mg/dL, but the two-hour postprandial is in the range of 140 to 199 mg/dL. Increased rates of obesity, hypertension, elevated triglycerides, and reduced high-density lipoprotein cholesterol levels often accompany IGT. Approximately one third of subjects with IGT progress to Type II diabetes.[4]

GOALS FOR GLYCEMIC CONTROL

There are specific goals that should be attained to achieve "good" glycemic control (Table 1).[5] It is no longer acceptable to have a hemoglobin HbA_{1c} of greater than 8 percent or a fasting plasma glucose (FPG) of greater than 140 mg/dL. In order to achieve these target values, it may be necessary to use multiple drug

Table 1. Glycemic guidelines of the American Diabetes Association

Biochemical index	Normal	Goal	Action suggested
Fasting/preprandial plasma glucose (mg/dl)	< 115	< 120	< 80 or > 140
Postprandial (mg/dl)	< 140	< 180	> 180
Bedtime glucose (mg/dl)	< 120	100–140	< 100 or > 160
Glycosylated hemoglobin*	< 6%	< 7%	> 8%

*Referred to a nondiabetic range of 4–6%.

therapy along with continued reinforcement of necessary lifestyle changes.

Recently, there has been a trend toward more aggressive management of people with diabetes. This stems from the conclusive clinical data that substantiate the benefit of tight glycemic control.[6-9] It is clear that achieving near normoglycemia in people with diabetes will prevent and slow the progression of the microvascular complications and reduce the risk of the macrovascular complications.[4-7] The recent availability of effective oral agents, acarbose, troglitazone, and metformin, provides alternatives to the standard therapy of oral sulfonylureas and insulin. Clinicians now have multiple agents with differing mechanisms and sites of action, allowing them to individualize the medication regimen and move toward normalizing the blood glucose levels.

The following case is representative of a typical patient with Type II diabetes. This patient presents with multiple disease states and various treatment issues that must be addressed. An indepth evaluation of the patient case will be presented along with recommendations for drug therapy modifications.

CASE PRESENTATION

BW is a 66-year-old male with a long-standing history of Type II diabetes. After numerous attempts at diet and exercise, the patient was placed on glyburide, which he has used for five years. The patient has recently been placed on glimepiride (Amaryl). BW comes to the clinic with complaints of increased thirst, urination, weakness, fatigue, blurred vision, and numbness/tingling in hands and feet.

The patient's medical history indicates that he had a myocardial infarction (MI) two years ago and has been diagnosed with diabetes for 15 years, hyperlipidemia for 2 years, and hypertension for 5 years. His father died of an MI at age 47, and his mother has diabetes. He has smoked one pack of cigarettes per day for 10 years and reports that he drinks a couple of beers per week. He is allergic to penicillin. His medications include Glimepiride (8 mg daily), atenolol (50 mg daily), and nicotinic acid (100 mg twice daily).

On physical examination, the patient is a 250 lb, 5'9" obese male in no apparent distress. His vital signs are as follows: blood pressure (mm Hg): 140/88, pulse: 81, respiratory rate (RR): 20, temperature: 98.5°F.

The patient has the following additional measures:

Sodium: 138 mEq/L (135 to 144); potassium: 4.5 mEq/L (3.5 to 5); fasting blood sugar: 189 mg/dL; HbA$_{1c}$: 10.5 percent; cholesterol: 200; low-density lipoprotein (LDL): 130; triglycerides: 225; high-density lipoprotein (HDL): 25; U/A 2+ glucose (–) ketones; carbon dioxide: 24 mEq/L (22 to 32); blood urea nitrogen: 21 mEq/L (10 to 20) serum creatinine 1.4 (.6 to 1.3).

Evaluate BW's Signs and Symptoms

The signs and symptoms that BW is having are suggestive of uncontrolled diabetes. The symptomatology of diabetes stems from the complex metabolic process involved in insulin production/release versus hormonal tissue requirements. Glucose concentrations become high after a meal secondary to decreased utilization and uptake of glucose by the cells. This is due to an absolute or relative lack of insulin. Fasting metabolism ensues, which triggers glycogenolysis and glyconeogenesis in the liver. As the blood glucose increases, the renal threshold is exceeded, and glucose spills into the urine, taking water with it. This causes an osmotic diuresis resulting in polyuria, polydipsia, fatigue, and weight loss.

BW is experiencing blurred vision and numbness and tingling in his extremities. These symptoms are suggestive of diabetic retinopathy and peripheral neuropathy.

Diabetic retinopathy, the most common complication of diabetes, is usually seen after 15 years. Approximately 700,000 people with diabetes have proliferative diabetic retinopathy.[10] The risk for glaucoma is 1.4 times more common in people with diabetes.[10] Diabetes is the leading cause of new cases of blindness in the United States with approximately 12,000 to 24,000 Americans becoming blind each year secondary to diabetes.[2,3]

Retinopathy is divided into two categories: (1) background (nonproliferative) or (2) proliferative. Nonproliferative retinopathy results from years of vascular insult caused by hyperglycemia-related damage to the capillary basement membrane. Proliferative retinopathy apparently involves a combination of hypoxia and the overproduction of sorbitol by the myoinositol pathway. There are microvascular effects resulting from diabetes-induced changes in the integrity of blood viscosity and of small blood vessels.[10] The risk of retinopathy and other vascular complications is significantly reduced when blood pressure and blood glucose are controlled. Retinal laser surgery can correct the retinopathy but should only be considered after tight control of blood glucose has failed.

About 60 to 70 percent of people with diabetes have mild to severe nerve damage, which can be diffuse or focal. Diffuse neuropathies include distal symmetrical polyneuropathy and autonomic neuropathies affecting the autonomic nervous system. Focal neuropathies may involve only one or a few nerve roots. The myoinositol system seems to be important in initiating a neuropathic reaction. Prolonged hyperglycemia alters the metabolic polyol pathway stimulating the production of sorbitol from glucose. Accumulation of sorbitol in nerve tissue decreases nerve conduction. The microvascular and macrovascular changes associated with hyperglycemia lead to hypoxia, which causes ischemic nerve injury; this also decreases nerve conduction velocity.[10] Signs and symptoms of neuropathy include pain in the lower extremities, paresthesias, decreased vibration sense, diabetic gastroparesis, and decreased tendon reflexes.

What Is Significant about the Patient's Medical History, Family History, Social History, and Physical Exam?

Family/Social history

There is a genetic basis for both Type I and Type II diabetes. A strong association exists between Type I diabetes and certain human leukocyte antigens (HLA) serotypes DR3 and DR4.[11] These are coded genes on the sixth chromosome. The presence of these antigens can cause an increased risk of Type I diabetes mellitus. Approximately 90 percent of Type II diabetic patients have a positive family history for diabetes.

Cardiovascular disease is two to four times more common in people with diabetes, and the risk of stroke is two and a half times higher in people with diabetes.[2] Coronary heart disease and other vascular diseases account for 1 million hospital admissions each year for people with diabetes. Since people with diabetes have a propensity toward developing cardiovascular disease, it is important that all risk factors, such as hypertension, hypercholesterolemia, smoking, and obesity are eliminated or reduced.

BW not only has a mother with diabetes but a father who died prematurely of an MI. A family history of coronary artery disease increases BW's risk of cardiovascular events. Ischemic heart disease is the leading cause of death in people with diabetes, and contributes to 40 percent of diabetes-related deaths, as shown in Figure 1. BW has several of these risk factors, which need to be addressed through counseling and lifestyle modifications and medications.

BW drinks "a couple of beers per week." The moderate consumption of alcohol will not affect blood glucose values in people with diabetes with "good" glycemic control. In people with diabetes, two or fewer alcohol beverages can be consumed daily but must be considered part of the meal plan. When calculating daily calories, alcohol should be substituted for a fat exchange. It is important to remember that alcohol may increase the risk of hypoglycemia in patients using antidiabetic agents (insulin and sulfonylureas).

What Factors Should Be Considered when Initiating Therapy in a Type II Diabetic Patient? What Is Significant Regarding BW's Current Drug Therapy?

The overall management of the Type II patient includes a combination of lifestyle modifications and pharmacologic agents. Both of these components of treatment must be maximized in order to achieve the target blood glucose value recommended by the American Diabetes Association (ADA). Not enough emphasis is placed on lifestyle changes and preventive health mea-

sures. Health care providers must give detailed information on diet and exercise to people with diabetes. People with diabetes must be encouraged to exercise regularly three to four times per week. A regular exercise program helps achieve an ideal body weight and improves the cardiovascular status of these Type II patients.

STEPS TO ACHIEVE GOOD GLYCEMIC CONTROL

First Step: Nonpharmacologic Treatment Modalities

The first step in the management of people with diabetes after diagnosis is to employ nonpharmacologic modalities, including diet, exercise, and lifestyle changes. These should be instituted three to six months before starting medication therapy. The exception to this rule is symptomatic patients with advanced disease (e.g., presence of microvascular and macrovascular complications at the time of diagnosis and a fasting plasma glucose of at least 250 mg/dL). These patients generally receive pharmacologic therapy at the time of diagnosis.

If, after three to six months of nonpharmacologic interventions, target values are not achieved, then one of the oral antidiabetic medi-

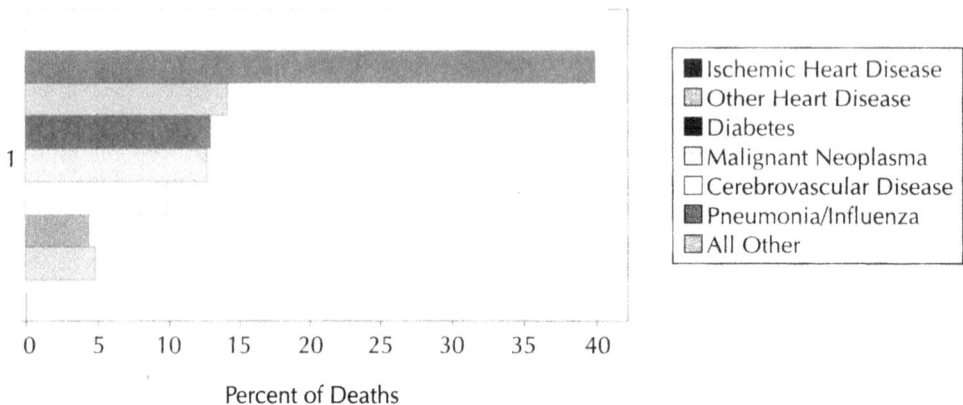

Figure 1. Approximate distribution of causes of death in people with diabetes, based on US studies. Source: Data from L.S. Geiss et al., "Mortality in Non-insulin Dependent Diabetes," in *Diabetes in America*, M.I. Harris et al., eds., pp. 236–237, © 1995, National Institutes of Health, National Institute of Diabetes and Digestive and Kidney Disease.

cations should be started. Drug therapy should begin with a single agent that is safe and effective with minimal weight gain and no hypoglycemia. Weight gain and hypoglycemia are not associated with use of acarbose or metformin as monotherapy but are seen with both the sulfonylureas and insulin.

Second Step: Monotherapy

The SFU can be used as first-line therapy in nonobese insulin-sensitive Type II patients. It is important that the cardiovascular status of the patient is assessed prior to beginning these agents. Studies have demonstrated an approximate 1 to 2 percent reduction in HbA1c.[12] BW is on glimepiride, which was approved November 30, 1995. It was Food and Drug Administration (FDA) approved for use in combination with insulin for Type II patients. The other SFUs have been used in combination with insulin. Glimepiride has a longer hypoglycemic effect than the other sulfonylureas.[13] The mechanism of action is similar to the other sulfonylureas.[13] The starting dose of glimepiride is 1 to 2 mg once daily, and the maintenance dose is 1 to 4 mg/day, with a maximum dose of 8 mg/day.

Since BW is already on 8 mg and has not achieved "target" values, another antidiabetic agent with a different mechanism of action should be added to the treatment regimen. Switching to another SFU generally will not provide any further reduction in blood glucose.

CASE PRESENTATION CONTINUED

The decision is made to add metformin 500 mg bid to BW's regimen, with a follow-up appointment in three months. The patient is instructed on home glucose monitoring, is given a blood glucose monitor, and is told to measure his blood sugars both fasting and after meals.

Third Step: Combination Therapy

If monotherapy does not achieve target values, then combination therapy should be initiated. If the patient has a fasting plasma glucose consistently greater than 200 mg/dL, then monotherapy usually will not achieve target values.[14] There have been studies showing beneficial effects of the sulfonylureas plus metformin[15–17] and the sulfonylureas plus acarbose.[18,19]

What Are the Pros and Cons of Metformin in This Patient? What Monitoring Parameters Would You Follow? How Would You Titrate the Metformin Dose?

Metformin can be used as the primary agent for the long-term treatment of Type II diabetes alone or in combination with sulfonylureas. It is most beneficial in obese, insulin-resistant patients. It may be a more rational choice than the sulfonylureas due to its beneficial effects on weight reduction, lack of hypoglycemic effects, and positive effect on lipid profiles.

BW has a serum creatinine at the upper limits of normal. Metformin is contraindicated in patients with renal impairment, liver disease alcoholism, intercurrent infection, and cardiopulmonary insufficiency. The manufacturer recommends that metformin should not be used if the serum creatinine is greater than 1.4 mg/dL in women and greater than 1.5 mg/dL in men. In patients with renal impairment or hypoxia, the risk of lactic acidosis secondary to metformin is increased. The dose of metformin should be titrated up slowly to eliminate gastrointestinal (GI) side effects. The initial dose is 500 mg daily and increased at no greater than weekly intervals up to 2,550 mg/day.

What Are the Therapeutic Considerations for the Other Medications that BW Is Receiving?

BW is receiving atenolol and nicotinic acid. Atenolol is a beta adrenergic antagonist that can cause severe hypoglycemic reactions in some individuals.[20] They can blunt the counter-regulatory effects of epinephrine that occur during hypoglycemic reactions, leading to a reduction in glycogenolysis. Most importantly, these agents attenuate the warning signs of hypoglycemia (i.e., tachycardia, hunger, tremor, irritability, and confusion). Sweating is one of the hypoglycemic signs that is not affected. In some patients, beta blockers may worsen glycemic control, adversely affect the lipid profile, and impair peripheral circulation. Since BW had a myocardial infarction two years ago, he is using atenolol for its cardioprotective effect. In these cases, most clinicians would continue the patient on the atenolol. A reduction in dosage may be warranted to maintain the cardioprotective effect and lessen the adverse affect on the diabetic state. Blood pressure should be monitored on an ongoing basis with a goal pressure of less than 130/85 mm Hg.[9] BW may require the addition of another antihypertensive agent to control his blood pressure once the atenolol is lowered.

BW is receiving nicotinic acid for his hyperlipidemia. In the diabetic patient, the goal is to lower the LDL cholesterol to less than 130 mg/dL.[9] If the patient has diabetes and coronary heart disease, the LDL cholesterol should be no more than 100 mg/dL, and the triglycerides no more than 200 mg/dL. A secondary goal of therapy is to increase the HDL cholesterol to greater than 35 mg/dL in men and 45 mg/dL in women.[9] The usual dose is 2 to 3 g/day. The current dosage of 100 mg twice a day is subtherapeutic. In Type II patients with diabetes, low HDL and high triglycerides are independent risk factors for cardiovascular disease.[21] It is therefore important to choose treatment that will affect both HDL and triglycerides. In nondiabetic patients, niacin and gemfibrozil would be effective agents. Unfortunately, niacin can increase insulin resistance and worsens glycemic control patients with diabetes.[21] In a recent study, 6 percent of established nondiabetic patients converted to clinical diabetes after two and a half years of niacin use. Gemfibrozil is not very effective in lowering LDL, and bile acid binding resins decrease LDL but can worsen triglycerides. In people with diabetes, the HMG-CoA reductase inhibitors are a good choice since they reduce total and LDL cholesterol and triglycerides and increase HDL cholesterol levels. These agents do not increase the blood glucose levels. At this point, the niacin should be discontinued, and a HMG-CoA reductase inhibitor should be initiated.

CASE PRESENTATION CONTINUED

BW returns to the clinic in three months. He has lost 15 lb. by adhering to his meal plan. He is feeling much better but complains of several hypoglycemic reactions. His BP is 142/90; pulse, 81; and weight, 230 lb. Other measures are as follows: Scr: 1.6 mg/dL; kidney panel (SMA 6): within normal limits (WNL) except Scr; liver function test (LFTs): WNL; FBS: 162 mg/dL; HbA1c: 9.0 percent; urine protein: 200 mg/24 hours. BW's blood glucose monitoring record is shown in Table 2.

What Changes in BW's Therapy Should Be Made at This Point?

Metformin was effective in lowering the fasting blood glucose and HbA1c in this patient. The serum creatinine has risen to 1.6 mg/dL, which

Table 2. Blood glucose (BG) monitoring record

Month October Date	Morning fasting BG	Breakfast (1 hour PPG) BG	Lunch (1 hour PPG) BG	Dinner (1 hour PPG) BG
4	160	172	220	242
5	168	176	188	224
6	172	182	208	238

Note: PPG = postprandial glucose.

precludes the continued use of metformin. Since BW has significant increases in postprandial blood glucose, acarbose would be a beneficial therapeutic choice.

Acarbose appears to be most beneficial in those patients with newly diagnosed diabetes or in those patients with high postprandial blood glucose (greater than 200 mg/dL) and normal or slightly elevated fasting blood glucose. It is both safe and effective with a positive effect on weight gain, insulin levels, and triglycerides. Studies have shown a significant reduction in postprandial blood sugars with a modest reduction in fasting plasma glucose.[22,23]

BW's blood pressure has increased slightly, and there is protein in his urine. Angiotensin converting enzyme (ACE) inhibitors are the drugs of choice for the treatment of hypertension in the diabetic patient. The ACE inhibitors have been found to reduce microalbuminuria, proteinuria, and hypoglycemic reactions since the absorption of sucrose and fructose is delayed. When sulfonylureas are used in combination with metformin or acarbose, a reduction in the sulfonylurea dose may be necessary.

How Would You Titrate the Acarbose Dose in This Patient?

It is very important to begin with a low dose of acarbose and increase the dose slowly. Slow titration of the medication has been found to improve the gastrointestinal intolerance seen with acarbose. The initial dose for acarbose is 25 mg at the first bite of the main meal. The dose can be increased after one to two weeks. For complete information on the dosing of acarbose, refer to Figure 2.

If Target Values Are Not Achieved with Orgal Agents, How Would You Initiate Insulin Therapy in This Patient?

Studies have shown that when insulin is added to the regimen of patients with sulfonylurea failure, a 1.7 percent reduction occurs in glycosylated hemoglobin. There appears to be better response

with combined treatment in patients who have been on insulin five years or less. Many clinicians advocate the use of bedtime insulin and daytime sulfonylureas (BIDs).[24] Evening insulin is beneficial based on the glycemic profile of the Type II diabetic patient. These patients tend to have the following:

- elevated fasting blood glucose with superimposed postprandial increase
- nadir in plasma glucose between 2 and 4 AM.
- "dawn phenomenon" before breakfast (increase in blood glucose at 5 AM due to secretion of growth hormone)

There are many ways of combining insulin and oral agents. The most popular regimens include the following:

- *Morning NPH and a long-acting oral sulfonylurea (glyburide) given one to two times a day.* With this regimen, the oral agent is used to prevent the overnight rise of hepatic glucose production and thereby control morning hyperglycemia.[21]
- *Bedtime NPH or Lente and a short-acting agent (glipizide).* With this regimen, the oral agent controls postprandial glucose excursions during the day, and the bedtime insulin reduces the glycemic rise that occurs from the "dawn phenomenon" and controls the fasting plasma glucose by suppressing excessive hepatic glucose output.[25]
- *Suppertime mixed insulin with daytime sulfonylureas (SMIDS).* In this regimen, split mixed or 70/30 insulin is given at suppertime with an oral agent given in the morning. SMIDS has been shown to achieve good fasting plasma glucose values with a reduction in the insulin dose required.[26]

The starting dose of NPH or Lente at bedtime is 10 to 20 U. The insulin dose should be increased every three to five days until the target fasting blood glucose is attained. Increases should be in increments of 0.025 to 0.075 U/kg.[27] In some insulin resistant Type II patients, large doses of intermediate acting insulin may be

Initial dosage: 25 mg tid (half of a scored 50-mg tablet)

Alternative initial dosage to minimize gastrointestinal side effects
Initial dosage: 25 mg once daily (half of a scored 50-mg tablet tid)
Gradually titrate to: 25 mg tid

For example:	Dose	Frequency	Duration*
	25mg	once daily[†]	1 to 2 weeks
	25 mg	bid	1 to 2 weeks
	25 mg	tid	4 to 8 weeks

Titrate to minimum maintenance dosage of 50 mg tid[‡]

Maintenance dosage: 50 mg tid to 100 mg tid
Maximum dosages: 50 mg tid for patients ≤ 132 lb.
                    100 mg tid for patients ≥ 132 lb.

*Based on European experience.
[†]Preferably taken with the evening meal.
[‡]Titration schedule should be individualized based on effectiveness and tolerance.

Figure 2. Dosing guidelines for acarbose (taken with the first bite of each main meal).

required (e.g., 60 to 80 U). If hypoglycemia develops on the combination therapy, the sulfonylurea dose should be decreased.

•   •   •

In summary, the following recommendations should be part of a pharmaceutical care plan for BW:

- Continue to counsel him on diet, exercise, and lifestyle modifications.
- Discontinue niacin and start an HMG-CoA reductase inhibitor to achieve goal values for LDL, triglycerides, and HDL.

- Consider reducing the dose of atenolol.
- Continue acarbose and titrate up to achieve "target" blood glucose and HbA1c values.
- Begin an ACE inhibitor since BW has evidence of proteinuria and needs to achieve a target blood pressure of less than 130/85 mm Hg.

All of these modifications in therapy should be done gradually. It is important to remember that diabetes is a chronic disease that requires a consistent and sustained approach toward improving the quality of life of people with diabetes.

REFERENCES

1. American Diabetes Association, *Diabetes 1996 Vital Statistics* (Alexandria, VA, 1996).

2. National Institute of Diabetes and Digestive and Kidney Diseases, *Diabetes Statistics.* NIH publication no. 96-3926 (Bethesda, MD, 1995).

3. National Diabetes Data Group, *Diabetes in America,* 2nd ed, NIH publication no. 95-1468 (Bethesda, MD: National Institutes of Health, 1995).

4. R. Holman, "Chairman's Introduction." *Diabetic Medicine* 13 (1996): S5.

5. American Diabetes Association, "Clinical Practice Recommendations Standards of Medical Care for Patients with Diabetes Mellitus," *Diabetes Care* 19, suppl. 1 (1996): S8–S15.

6. The Diabetes Control and Complications Trial Research Group, "The effect of Intensive Treatment of Diabetes on the Development and Progression of Long Term Complications in Insulin-dependent-diabetes Mellitus," *New England Journal of Medicine* 329 (1993): 977–986.

7. Y. Ohkubo et al., "Intensive Insulin Therapy Prevents the Progression of Diabetic Microvascular Complica-

tions in Japanese Patients with Non-insulin Dependent Diabetes Mellitus: A Radomized Prospective 6-Year Study," *Diabetes Research Clinical Practice* 28 (1995): 103–117.

8. J. Kususisto et al., "NIDDM and Its Metabolic Control Predict Coronary Heart Disease in Elderly Subjects," *Diabetes* 43 (1993): 960–967.

9. United Kingdom Prospective Diabetes Study 16, "Overview of 6 Years' Therapy of Type II Diabetes: A Progressive Disease," *Diabetes* 44 (1995): 1,249–1,258.

10. C.F. Steil, "Chronic Complications of Diabetes," *American Pharmacy* NS31 (1991): 37–44.

11. W.A. Simon, "Can IDDM Be Prevented?" *US Pharmacist* (1995): H3–H9.

12. J.R. White, "The Pharmacologic Management of Patients with Type II Diabetes Mellitus in the Era of New Oral Agents and Insulin Analogs." *Diabetes Spectrum* 9 (1996): 227–234.

13. "Glimepiride: Drugs of the Future," 17, no. 9 (1992): 774–778.

14. C.J. Bailey, and R.C. Turner, "Metformin," *New England Journal of Medicine* 334 (1996): 574–579.

15. R.A. DeFronzo, and A.M. Goodman, "Efficacy of Metformin in Patients with Non-Insulin-dependent Diabetes Mellitus," *New England Journal of Medicine* 333 (1995): 541–549.

16. L.S. Hermann et al., "Therapeutic Comparison of Metformin and Sulfonylureas, Alone and in Various Combinations: A Double-blind Controlled Study," *Diabetes Care* 17 (1994): 1,100–1,109.

17. G.M. Reaven et al., "Combined Metformin-sulfonylurea Treatment of Patients with Non-insulin Dependent Diabetes in Fair to Poor Glycemic Control," *Journal of Clinical Endocrinology and Metabolism* 74 (1992): 1,020–1,026.

18. R.F. Coniff et al., "Multicenter, Placebo-Controlled Trial Comparing Acarbose (BAY g5421) with Placebo, Tolbutamide and Tolbutamide plus Acarbose in Non-insulin-dependent Diabetes Mellitus," *American Journal of Medicine* 98 (1995): 443–451.

19. S. Vannasaeng et al., "Effects of Alpha-glucosidase Inhibitor (Acarbose) Combined with Sulfonylurea or Sulfonylurea and Metformin in Treatment of Non-insulin-dependent Diabetes Mellitus." *Journal of the Medical Association of Thailand* 78 (1995): 578–584.

20. J.R. White et al., "Drug Interactions in Diabetic Patients," *Postgraduate Medicine* 93 (1993): 131–139.

21. A.J. Garber, "Diabetes and Heart Disease: A New Strategy for Managing Lipid Disorders." *Geriatrics* 8 (1993): 34–41.

22. J. Hoffman, and M. Spengler, "Efficacy of 24 Week Monotherapy with Acarbose, Glibenclamide or Placebo in NIDDM Patients," *Diabetes Care* 17 (1994): 561–566.

23. R.F. Coniff et al., "Long-term Efficacy and Safety of Acarbose in the Treatment of Obese Subjects with Non-insulin-dependent Diabetes Mellitus," *Archives of Internal Medicine* 154 (1994): 2,442–2,448.

24. A.L. Peters, and M.B. Davidson, "BIDS Therapy for Treatment of NIDDM: Effectiveness and Predictors (if Any) of Success," *Diabetes Spectrum* 7 (1994): 152–158.

25. L.C. Groop et al., "Combined Insulin-sulfonylurea Therapy in Treatment of NIDDM," *Diabetes Care* 13, suppl. 3 (1990): 47–52.

26. C.R. Garrison, and M.C. Riddle, "Evening Insulin Therapy for Type II Diabetes," *Practical Diabetology* 9 (1990): 1–5.

27. D.F. Brown, and T.W. Jackson, "Diabetes: Tight Control in a Comprehensive Treatment Plan." *Geriatrics* 49 (1994): 24–36.

PART IV

Disease Management and Economics

Disease management is a term of recent vintage that describes a more global approach to minimizing the cost and impact of disease. Because the term is so recent in origin, there is no benchmark definition. However, the authors in this section define many of the boundaries of the term and its use.

The chapter by Cooke describes the methods used to create care plans and pathways. These pathways and tools are used to develop patient management strategies that are then examined by using outcomes assessment methodologies. Although there are few disease management programs in diabetes care, the opportunities to create value by using this methodology are greater. Monaghan and Monaghan examine the current state of pharmaceutical care in diabetes management. Their focus demonstrates the continuing need for pharmacists to design systems that provide pharmaceutical care to patients and documents the activities, interventions, and education that support the improvements.

Finally, Pathak and Burke examine the societal and economic impacts of diabetes mellitus. Their approach examines the methods that can be used to determine the cost and impact of patient care interventions in diabetes. They also examine the usefulness of several methods for determining the value of outcomes. Diabetes mellitus is an excellent model for assessing the impact of disease on functionality and quality of life. The impact of pharmacists on patient care outcomes in diabetes remains to be determined; however, we have developed an excellent clinical database and practice role from which to embark.

CHAPTER 13

Disease State Management in Diabetes Care

Catherine E. Cooke, PharmD

Diabetes affects over 16 million Americans. Caring for patients with diabetes requires extensive health care resources. Managed care organizations must utilize resources cost-effectively to survive in the health care industry. A disease state management program for diabetes may enable the managed care organization to meet its goal of providing cost-effective quality health care while meeting regulatory standards. The National Committee for Quality Assurance (NCQA) which accredits managed care organizations and provides information on performance, grants accreditation status to managed care organizations and reports favorable comparisons with competing managed care organizations. Key words: *diabetes mellitus, disease state management, managed care organization, NCQA, HEDIS*

Over 16 million people in the United States currently suffer from diabetes. The consequences of diabetes can be financially and emotionally debilitating. From a health-system perspective, caring for these patients requires an enormous amount of resources. Managed care organizations are designed to provide quality health care in a cost-effective manner while meeting industry standards. Although several ways exist to help achieve the managed care organization's goal, disease management programs may be a cost-effective method to care for patients with diabetes. A successful disease state management program in diabetes care should achieve optimal therapeutic, economic, and humanistic outcomes. This article focuses on the value and use of disease management programs in diabetes care.

MANAGED CARE

Managed care is a term which describes the way care is offered, delivered, and paid for.

Managed care organizations can be defined as integrated health systems offering health care services for a pre-paid fee. Several different types of managed care organizations exist, e.g., health maintenance organizations (HMO), and preferred provider organizations (PPO).[1] HMOs can be one of several types as well: staff, group, independent practice association (IPA), and network. The type of managed care organization determines the way care is delivered. In a staff model HMO, the health care providers are salaried by the managed care organization and provide direct patient care to covered members. In an IPA, either a group of physicians within an office or solo practitioners can contract with the managed care organization to provide care for patients with health care coverage from that managed care organization. However, these practitioners, unlike those salaried by the managed care organization, are able to care for patients with other insurance coverage. Increasingly, health care practitioners in various health care fields such as medicine, pharmacy, physical therapy, and nursing are involved with managed care. The penetration of managed care organizations differs by geographic region. Although penetration is greatest in the western United States, over 20% of the population in the continental United States have managed care as their health insurance.[2]

The overall goal of managed care organizations is to achieve quality health care in a cost-effective manner while meeting industry standards. Pharmacy has been important in helping managed care organizations achieve this goal. Traditionally, the pharmacy budget has been carved out and pharmacists have been effective at reducing drug expenditures. However, the industry is shifting away from looking solely at the cost of pharmaceutical products. From a health system perspective, it may be cost-effective to use a more expensive medication which reduces hospitalizations or emergency department visits. Using a less costly medication which is less effective in reducing other more expensive health care expenditures would be short-sighted. However, for this approach to succeed, the pharmacy budget must be integrated into total budget costs. Disease state management is a concept that embraces a comprehensive approach to caring for patients with a particular disease while considering the total costs of care for that disease.

DISEASE STATE MANAGEMENT

Disease state management is a comprehensive integrated approach to patient care and reimbursement.[3] There are two goals of disease state management programs. The first is to improve patient care. Therapeutic and humanistic outcomes are measured to ensure that this first goal is achieved. The second goal is to utilize resources efficiently while caring for patients with a particular disease. Economic parameters (e.g., cost of outpatient visits, hospitalizations, emergency department visits, drug therapy) are used to determine the use of resources for that disease.

Typically, diseases which are targeted in disease state management programs have several common characteristics (see the box titled,

Common Characteristics of Diseases Suitable for Disease State Management Programs).[4] Diabetes is a chronic disease which can result in serious sequelae with significant costs if not treated appropriately. There is enough medical literature to support consensus on how best to manage patients with diabetes from a therapeutic outcomes perspective.[5,6] Pharmacoeconomics can determine which treatment regimens are more cost-effective than others, and patient quality-of-life can be measured with various instruments such as the validated Medical Outcomes Study Short Form 36 (MOS SF-36).[7] Currently over 45 percent of HMOs in the United States have implemented disease management initiatives in diabetes care.[8]

The elements of disease state management programs include clinical practice guidelines, formulary modifications, educational interventions, and outcomes assessment.[9]

Clinical Practice Guidelines

The first element of a disease state management program is developing clinical practice guidelines. Algorithms, care plans, care maps, and critical pathways are synonyms for clinical practice guidelines. Clinical practice guidelines have been developed by government organizations (e.g., the Agency for Health Care Policy and Research [AHCPR]) and professional pharmacy organiza-

---

Common Characteristics of Diseases Suitable for Disease State Management Programs

1. Chronic disease with high prevalence
2. Significant costs associated with treatment of the disease or its complications
3. Treatment usually involves choices of therapy (lifestyle modifications, pharmacological, surgical)
4. Consensus of appropriate treatment protocols
5. Defined clinical outcomes of efficacy and toxicity

tions (e.g., American Pharmaceutical Association). Clinical practice guidelines are developed to standardize decision-making for the majority of patients who fit certain specified criteria. Clinical practice guidelines for appropriate screening, prevention, and treatment for patients with diabetes have been developed by the American Diabetic Association.[5] Guidelines incorporate all aspects of patient care from a patient walking into the office, screening for diabetes, and diagnosing a patient with diabetes to chronic care of that patient. Specific information on the history, physical exam, patient education, and therapy should be detailed. Care during hospitalizations, emergency department visits, and pancreas transplants may also be included when developing clinical practice guidelines.

Pharmacists are integral in the design, implementation, and success of disease management programs. Pharmacists, especially community pharmacists who have access to large numbers of patients, can help screen for diabetes. The clinical practice guidelines may help determine who to screen. High-risk patients should be screened. These include the following patients:

- American Indian, Hispanic, or African American races
- those with a positive family history
- age ≥45 years
- obesity (greater than 20% over ideal body weight)
- patients with hypertension or hyperlipidemia (cholesterol ≥240 mg/dL or triglycerides ≥250 mg/dL)
- symptomatic patients (polyuria, polydipsia, polyphagia)
- women with a history of gestational diabetes or babies weighing greater than 9 lbs at birth[5]

For patients with any of these criteria, a fasting plasma glucose test can be performed in the pharmacy. If the patient's glucose level is elevated (for non-pregnant adults, >115 mg/dL fasting), the pharmacist can refer the patient to the physician for a glucose tolerance test.

Following the diagnosis of diabetes, the pharmacist can help determine appropriate therapy for the patient. Pharmacists can educate patients about lifestyle modifications and reinforce healthy lifestyle practices at each visit. Once a patient has failed lifestyle modifications, pharmacotherapy may be required. There are several choices for initial therapy. Although insulin is considered an option for initial therapy, sulfonylureas, metformin, and acarbose are preferred due to patient acceptability, compliance and potential risks associated with insulin therapy. Comparative reductions in HbA$_{1c}$ (glycosylated hemoglobin) are about 1.5 percent–2 percent for sulfonylureas and metformin and 0.5 percent–1 percent for acarbose.[5] To determine the most cost-effective initial therapy, four aspects need to be considered: 1) cost of the agent, 2) efficacy, 3) toxicity, and 4) patient acceptance.

Currently there is no consensus as to which class of agents is preferable for initial monotherapy. Patient variables will dictate the choice of one agent over another. Pharmacists must use clinical judgment to recommend the appropriate therapy for the individual patient. While clinical practice guidelines are intended to provide guidance for the care of the majority of patients with the disease, individual patient characteristics should be considered when determining optimal therapy.

Formulary Modifications

Managed care organizations usually have drug formularies, a list of the drug products which are approved for use by their members. In other words, a formulary is a list of medications for which the managed care organization subsidizes the cost. Typically, patients have to pay only a co-pay which may be determined by the status of the drug product. For example, generic medications are usually associated with lower co-pays than their trade name counterpart.

In disease state management, the formulary recommendations for the particular disease will be based on the clinical practice guidelines. The clinical practice guidelines may determine that therapy with sulfonylureas is appropriate initial therapy for the patient with Type II diabetes. However, allowing all sulfonylureas on the formulary would not be economically advantageous. If one or two sulfonylureas were chosen for formulary inclusion, the managed care organization could either purchase these agents at a discount or receive a manufacturer's rebate secondary to increased volume. The four factors as mentioned in the *Clinical Practice Guidelines* section above apply to determining the most cost-effective agent within a class. If glipizide, glyburide, and tolbutamide are determined to be the only sulfonylureas that are appropriate for patients with Type II diabetes, then these will be the only approved sulfonylureas on the formulary. Patients are able to receive other sulfonylureas, however, they will incur a greater expense for these products. The same principles hold true for deciding which insulin product should be on the formulary. Metformin and acarbose are the only acceptable agents in their respective classes, and do not compete for formulary inclusion. When other safe and effective biguanides are available, metformin will compete for a place on the formulary.

Educational Interventions

In order for disease state management program goals to be met, physicians and other prescribers must be educated about these goals, clinical practice guidelines, and formulary products available to them. If health care providers are unaware of this information, they may not be treating patients with diabetes in a manner which will achieve optimal therapeutic, economic, and humanistic outcomes. Suggestions for successful education are to involve health care providers in clinical practice guideline development, distribute draft guidelines for feedback, provide one-on-one educational sessions, and continuously re-evaluate the guidelines and the disease state management process. Reporting individual assessment back to the provider has been shown to encourage adherence to the guidelines.[10]

Outcomes Assessment

Outcomes assessment is necessary to determine whether the disease management program is making a difference. Three outcomes used to evaluate care for the patient with diabetes are: therapeutic, economic, and humanistic outcomes (see Table 1). Therapeutic parameters include HbA_{1c}. Based on the Diabetes Control and Complications Trial (DCCT) and the Diabetes Care consensus statement, a desirable HbA_{1c} would be <7 mg/dL.[5,6] Measuring HbA_{1c} would enable the managed care organization to determine how many patients have their diabetes under adequate control. Although the goal in treating diabetes is to decrease morbidity and mortality, using surrogate measures may be more practical. Blood glucose and HbA_{1c} have

Table 1. Therapeutic, economic, and humanistic parameters used to evaluate outcomes

Therapeutic	Economic ($$)	Humanistic
HbA_{1c}	Hospitalizations	Quality-of-life
Blood glucose	Surgeries/procedures: amputations	MOS SF-36
Fasting	Emergency department visits	TyPE specific
Post-prandial	Pharmacotherapy/diabetic supplies	Patient satisfaction
Retinopathy	Physician/provider visits	
Nephropathy	Laboratory/X-ray/ECG tests	
Scr/BUN		
Neuropathy		
Cardiovascular disease		

Note: ECG, electrocardiogram.

correlated with microvascular complications such as retinopathy, nephropathy, and neuropathy. Therefore, achieving goal HbA1c levels may lead us to believe that we are decreasing morbidity associated with diabetes. However, HbA1c has not been shown to correlate with macrovascular complications (e.g., atherosclerotic heart disease).[6] That is why a disease state management program for patients with diabetes would include cardiovascular risk reduction practices (e.g., lifestyle modifications, controlling hypertension and hyperlipidemia). As reduction in HbA1c does not correlate with reduction in macrovascular complications from diabetes, cardiovascular morbidity and mortality must be measured. Economic parameters evaluate the use of resources and costs associated with their use. Typically, the costs of hospitalizations, emergency department visits, and surgeries/procedures will determine the cost of caring for patients with diabetes. Although these occurrences may be infrequent, the costs associated with one hospitalization or surgery are tremendous. However, all parameters need to be included to determine cost-effective diabetes care. Humanistic parameters include measuring patient quality-of-life and satisfaction. Often times, patient satisfaction surveys are developed internally (e.g., within the managed care organization). Several instruments are available to measure quality-of-life. The SF-36 is intended to measure overall health status and is not disease specific. Quality-of-life questionnaires which have been designed for particular disease states may be more useful in disease state management.

"REGULATORY" AGENCIES

The National Committee for Quality Assurance (NCQA) is an organization which evaluates managed care organizations.[11-13] The two main func-

tions of NCQA are to accredit managed care organizations and to measure and report on their performance according to standardized measures. The NCQA uses a set of standardized performance measures called Health Employer Data Information Set (HEDIS) to evaluate managed care organizations. A helpful analogy is NCQA is to managed care organizations what the Joint Committee on the Accreditation of Hospital Organizations is to hospitals.

The requirements for meeting NCQA standards are driving some managed care organizations to incorporate disease state management programs. Patient satisfaction surveys and quality-of-life issues need to be addressed for NCQA to grant accreditation status.[14] The survival of managed care organizations is probably going to be dependent partly on successful disease state management programs.

Currently, over half of the managed care organizations in the United States have gone through accreditation. Of those, 80% have received accreditation for at least one year. This information is reported publicly to help patients determine the quality of different managed care organizations.

CONCLUSION

Disease state management is one way in which managed health care plans can demonstrate to NCQA and the population that they are providing better diabetes care. The four components which need to be considered for successful disease management programs are the practice guidelines, formulary modifications, educational interventions, and outcomes assessment. Diabetes disease state management may be one way of improving the care of patients who have diabetes in a cost effective manner.

REFERENCES

1. C. Cooke, and M. Wilson, "Managed Care Organizations: Today and Tomorrow," *American Druggist* 211, no. 1 (1994): 67–74.

2. "Trend of the Month: Managed Care in the United State." *Drug Benefit Trends* 7, no. 7 (1995): 6.

3. R.S. Hadsall, and L.J. Sargent, "Disease State Manage-

ment," in *A Pharmacist's Guide to Principles and Practices of Managed Care Pharmacy*, ed. S.M. Ito and S. Blackburn (Alexandria, Virginia: Foundation for Managed Care Pharmacy, 1995), 163–68.

4. G. Muirhead, "Disease Management: Threat or opportunity for pharmacy?" *Drug Topics* 139, no. 15 (August 7, 1995): 50, 52, 54, 56, 59.

5. American Diabetes Association: Clinical Practice Recommendations 1996, *Diabetes Care* 19, supplement 1 (1996): S1–S118.

6. The Diabetes Control and Complications Trial Research Group, "The Effect of Intensive Treatment of Diabetes on the Development and Progression of Long-term Complications in Insulin-dependent Diabetes Mellitus," *New England Journal of Medicine* 329 (1993): 977–986.

7. C. Jenkinson, L. Wright, and A. Coulter, "Criterion Validity and Reliability of the SF-36 in a Population Sample," *Quality of Life Research* 3, no. 1 (1994): 7–12.

8. Trend of the Month: Disease Management Initiatives Succeeding in HMOs, *Drug Benefit Trends,* 8, no. 12, 1996, 8.

9. E.P. Armstrong, "Disease State Management and its Influence on Health Systems Today," *Drug Benefit Trends* 7 (1996): 18–29.

10. J.M. Schectman, N.K. Kanwal, W.S. Schroth, and E.G. Elinsky, "The Effect of an Education and Feedback Intervention on Group-model and Network-model Health Maintenance Organization Physician Prescribing Behavior," *Medical Care* 33, no. 2 (1995): 139–144.

11. J.K. Iglehart, "The National Committee for Quality Assurance." *New England Journal of Medicine* 335, no. 13 (1996): 995–999.

12. R.H. Brook, E.A. McGlynn, and P.D. Cleary, "Part 2: Measuring Quality of Care," *New England Journal of Medicine* 335, no. 13 (1996): 966–970.

13. M.A. Bloomberg et al., "Development of Clinical Indicators for Performance Measurement and Improvement: An HMO/purchaser Collaborative Effort." *Joint Commission Journal on Quality Improvement* 19 (1993): 586–595.

14. The National Committee for Quality Assurance. 1996. *1996 Reviewer Guidelines for Accreditation of Managed Care Organizations* (effective April 1996 through March 1997).

CHAPTER 14

Are Pharmacists and Pharmaceutical Care Having an Impact on Diabetes?

Maura J. Monaghan, PharmD, MBA and Michael S. Monaghan, PharmD

This study sought to identify pharmacy services offered to patients with diabetes and demonstrate patients receiving pharmaceutical care services had better glucose control as measured by laboratory values and medication compliance. Two hundred randomly selected patients with diabetes were identified from a pharmacy benefits manager's database. Their pharmacists were mailed a survey requesting information concerning morbidity risk factors, concomitant disease states, concomitant medications, diabetes pharmacotherapy, blood glucose concentrations, and percent hemoglobin A_{1c} values. Information concerning diabetes cognitive services offered was also requested. A statistically significant correlation between diabetes cognitive services and improved disease control was not demonstrated secondarily to the small number of responses returned with glucose control information. Our results indicate pharmacists must improve documentation of their services and the impact these interventions have on disease control in order to prepare for reimbursement for cognitive services. Key words: *cognitive services, diabetes mellitus, documentation*

INTRODUCTION

In today's marketplace, health care providers strive to deliver state-of-the-art patient care which is also cost-effective. Pharmacists may play an invaluable role in this endeavor since new and investigational medical treatments often involve expensive pharmaceuticals. Being experts in drug use and capable of using physical assessment as a monitoring parameter, pharmacists are a cost-effective answer to the question of who should monitor drug therapy in the emerging managed care environment. Such a practice would fulfill the challenge offered through the expansion of pharmacy practice away from a purely distributive role, namely pharmaceutical care.

Pharmaceutical care, incorporating the use of a treatment plan for the purpose of achieving pa-tient-specific outcomes which will positively affect one's quality of life, is well-defined elsewhere.[1-3] Pharmacists generally provide pharmaceutical care through the provision of cognitive services. Cognitive services may be defined as any action taken by a pharmacist, for the patient's benefit, not directly associated with the dispensing of a pharmaceutical product. Factors which motivate pharmacists to deliver pharmaceutical care are financial, ethical, and legal incentives. When a financial incentive or reimbursement is offered, pharmacists are more likely to offer cognitive services.[4,5] This suggests most community practitioners are unable to depend more on fees derived from cognitive (i.e., pharmacy) services than those

This work was made possible through an educational grant supplied by the Pharmacia and Upjohn Pharmaceutical Company.

129

derived from dispensing a product. Thus, the dilemma: do pharmacists provide comprehensive pharmaceutical care for ethical and professional reasons, with the hope that future payors will realize the positive impact on overall health care expenditures and financially reimburse for pharmacy services? Or, should pharmacists wait for the payor to offer financial incentives for pharmaceutical care delivery before providing these patient services? Regardless, pharmacists must document their cognitive interventions and, if possible, the impact these interventions are having on disease control.

The concept of pharmaceutical care continues to be a topic for discussion in academic and professional forums. For more than 20 years, the literature has discussed pharmacy care as a means of targeting specific disease states, such as diabetes.[6] Published surveys reveal pharmacists believe patients want and need pharmaceutical care. However, respondents were not confident when addressing three areas: 1) physician cooperation with the delivery of pharmaceutical care, 2) their current knowledge base, and 3) assessment of laboratory parameters required for therapeutic drug monitoring.[7] These concerns represent some of the barriers to pharmaceutical care delivery. Are these barriers preventing the delivery of pharmaceutical care?

We recently surveyed a random selection of pharmacies belonging to a pharmacy provider network in a rural state. The pharmacy network contains 47% chain pharmacies and 53% independently owned pharmacies. The purpose of the survey was to identify specific pharmacy services offered to patients with diabetes and demonstrate patients receiving pharmaceutical care services had better glucose control as measured by laboratory values (e.g., fasting blood glucose concentration and percent hemoglobin A_{1c}) and medication compliance. Our intent was to use the results as a marketing tool for a diabetes management program and generate reimbursement for pharmacy services. The results of this survey are not conclusive; rather they suggest pharmacists must improve documentation of services and the impact these interventions have on disease control.

METHODS AND MATERIALS

Patients with diabetes were identified from a pharmacy benefits manager's (PBM) database. All patients receiving an oral sulfonylurea were considered eligible. Of the 7,367 patients identified, 200 were randomly selected. A table of random numbers was used for patient selection. The dispensing pharmacist was mailed a survey (Appendix A) which identified the study patient by name. No constraints were placed on the type of patient, prescriber, PBM client, or type of pharmacy during the randomization process. After one month, a second copy of the survey was sent to nonrespondents. After two more months, each nonrespondent was phoned and requested to complete and return the survey.

The survey requested information concerning patient demographics, morbidity risk factors, concomitant disease states, concomitant medications, diabetes, pharmacotherapy, blood glucose concentrations (fasting or home blood glucose readings), and percent hemoglobin A_{1c} values (HgbA$_{1c}$). If pharmacists provided information concerning blood glucose concentrations or HgbA$_{1c}$, they were asked to identify the source of this information. Additionally, the survey requested information concerning cognitive services offered which were specific for patients with diabetes. Pharmacists were paid $15 for their time and effort.

Returned surveys were tabulated for data analysis. All patient medication profiles were reviewed to determine survey accuracy; all information was verified by claims transactions. Specifically, risk factors and dosage changes identified by the pharmacist were verified to determine the accuracy of pharmacists' histories. Also, an attempt to identify differences between chain and independent pharmacies was made in medication compliance rates and patient loyalty as determined by pharmacy use during the past six months.

Statistical analysis consisted of descriptive data concerning diabetes cognitive services offered and laboratory parameters monitored. Also, chain versus independent pharmacies were compared using a chi-square analysis to determine if a difference existed in frequency of cognitive services offered. Further, a Mann-Whitney U test was performed to determine if there was a difference in pharmacist data (year graduated) between the groups. A correlation coefficient was calculated to determine the significance of the relationship between cognitive services offered and glucose control indicated by laboratory parameters. Statistical significance was defined as $p < 0.05$.

RESULTS

Of the 200 patients identified, only 193 were used. Seven were eliminated due to patients moving out of state, changing employment, or death. Of the 193 surveys mailed, only 101 (52.3 percent) were returned, even after two contacts. However, because of incomplete responses, only 70 were evaluable secondary to missing data. According to phone contact with nonresponders, reasons for returning incomplete surveys included: patient not a regular client, patient confidentiality concerns, pharmacists unable to obtain information, and pharmacist did not have time to fill out the survey due to OBRA '90 requirements. A number of surveys were returned with only pharmacy demographics and did not provide the requested patient information.

Table 1 shows survey response rates, percent of evaluable surveys, medication compliance rates, and loyalty rates by pharmacy type (chain versus independent). Independent pharmacies had a higher survey return rate. But of those returned, independent pharmacies had a lower rate of evaluable surveys. Medication compliance rates favored chain pharmacies while patient loyalty favored independent pharmacies. A statistical difference was seen only in the pharmacists' year of graduation.

Table 2 contains the frequency of cognitive services delivered. Most pharmacies provide compliance counseling in addition to diabetes medication counseling. However, few monitor markers of disease control such as blood glucose concentrations (e.g., home blood glucose records or fasting plasma glucose) or HgbA1c. When these values were known, they were most often obtained from the patient, followed by the physician, nurse, and last from the pharmacy's own profiles. The provision of written material, specific to diabetes, occurred greater than 50% of the time. There was no significant difference between diabetes cognitive services offered by chain and independent pharmacies. Independent pharmacies tended to offer more services, but statistical significance could not be determined secondary to the small numbers offering these services. The primary purpose of the study, a significant correlation between diabetes cognitive services and improved disease control, was not demonstrated. Only 17 surveys were returned with glucose control information.

DISCUSSION

The American Diabetes Association (ADA) revised standards of medical care[8] stress four areas of cognitive services which pharmacists can

Table 1. Differences in survey response rates, medication compliance, patient loyalty, and year of graduation by type of pharmacy

	Chain Pharmacy	Independent Pharmacy
Number of surveys mailed	86	107
Response rate	33.7%	66.4%
Percent of evaluable surveys	82.8%	64.8%
A medication compliance rate in evaluable population	52.5%	47.5%
Loyalty rates in evaluable population	88.8%	95.3%
Average year of graduation from pharmacy school*	1981	1974

*$p < 0.05$

Table 2. Performance of cognitive services as they relate to diabetes by type of pharmacy

Cognitive Service	Number of Chains Providing Service (%)	Number of Independents Providing Service (%)	Total Number Providing Service (%)
Compliance counseling	23 (95.8)	42 (91.3)	65 (92.9)
Medication counseling	24 (100)	43 (93.5)	67 (95.7)
Lifestyle counseling	21 (87.5)	41 (89.1)	62 (88.6)
Perform blood glucose screenings	2 (8.3)	7 (15.2)	9 (12.8)
Provide diabetes education material	11 (45.8)	33 (71.7)	44 (62.8)
Monitor blood glucose	1 (4.2)	10 (21.7)	11 (15.7)
Monitor percent hemoglobin A_{1c}	5 (20.8)	1 (2.2)	6 (8.6)

provide to aid in the treatment of people with diabetes: 1) patient education, 2) continuity of care, 3) frequent patient contact, and 4) referral to specialists when necessary. The vast majority of people with diabetes are treated by general practitioners and not diabetes specialists.[9] Because of this, some patients may be lost to follow-up. Pharmacists, being the health care practitioners most accessible to the public, can act as a safety net and ensure a continuity of care for the patient with diabetes. Pharmacists can review problems that may have occurred since the last physician visit and aid in correcting them or refer the person on to the physician. The ADA recommends frequent physician visitations. Because physicians are not always available, the pharmacist may be able to assist patients at times when the physician is unavailable, if only to answer questions and serve as a patient advocate. Also, pharmacists can stress therapeutic compliance with each visit, maintaining therapeutic integrity. Lastly, pharmacists can remind patients to see the ophthalmologist, dietetic counselor, podiatrist, and dentist when recommended.

Documentation of the above cognitive services and how these services are impacting disease control will be important in justifying financial reimbursement from third-party payors. The best means of assessing how cognitive services impact disease control is through the use of monitoring parameters which assess disease control, such as HgbA1c.

HgbA1c reflect the average blood glucose concentration over the previous two to three months.[10] In persons without diabetes, normal values usually range between 3 percent and 6 percent, while people with uncontrolled diabetes can have values 3 times as high. Generally, a 1 percent change in HgbA1c reflects a 25–35 mg/dL change in average blood glucose concentration.[11] Therefore, a HgbA1c of 7 percent corresponds to an average blood glucose concentration of about 150 mg/dL and a HgbA1c of 9 percent corresponds to an average glucose concentration of around 210 mg/dL over the previous 2–3 months. What this means, as demonstrated by the Diabetes Control and Complications Trial,[12] is a person with a HgbA1c of 7 percent is much less likely to develop long-term diabetes complications than one with a HgbA1c of 9 percent.[13] The average cost of a HgbA1c measurement is approximately $30. Thus, HgbA1c is an inexpensive means of objectively assessing a person's risk for the development of diabetes complications.[14] HgbA1c is probably the best mode for pharmacists to use in assessing the effectiveness of overall treatment.

We found that diabetes cognitive services offered by chain and independent pharmacies did not differ significantly. Neither group recorded blood glucose concentrations nor HgbA1c with frequency. This may be due to the pharmacist's lack of accessibility to this data or due to few patients knowing their HgbA1c or willing to monitor/share their home blood glucose values. In this study, chain pharmacists graduated more recently than those working in independent pharmacies. Chain pharmacies also returned fewer but more evaluable surveys. The more complete surveys from chain pharmacies could be due to the younger pharmacists working. One explanation for the more complete surveys coming from chains may be that younger pharmacists document more or are aware of the importance of documenting activities and therefore completed the forms more fully.

CONCLUSIONS

Our results indicate that if pharmacists are providing cognitive diabetes services, they are not documenting their interventions. It is imperative that as pharmacists, we make an effort to docu-ment interventions and correlate these services with disease control measurements (blood glucose concentrations and HgbA1c). Managed care organizations will reimburse the most cost-effective health care professional documenting his or her impact on the disease state in question. The authors believe most pharmacists are offering diabetes cognitive services. But without documentation, we pharmacists will not be reimbursed for services other than dispensing. The profession has been challenged to change its role as healthcare providers; we are summoned to take responsibility for patient outcomes. Because of our knowledge of drug therapy and our accessibility, diabetes is an ideal disease with which to implement our new practice model—pharmaceutical care. Pharmacists must increase the documentation of their services and the impact of these services if we hope to be reimbursed for cognitive interventions.

REFERENCES

1. C.D. Hepler, and L.M. Strand, "Opportunities and Responsibilities in Pharmaceutical Care," *American Journal of Hospital Pharmacy* 47 (1990): 533–543.

2. R.P. Penna, "Pharmaceutical Care: Pharmacy's Mission for the 1990s," *American Journal of Hospital Pharmacy* 47 (1990): 543–549.

3. L.M. Strand et al., "Integrated Patient-specific Model of Pharmacy Practice," *American Journal of Hospital Pharmacy* 47 (1990): 550–554.

4. M.J. Miller, and B.G. Ortmeier, "Factors Influencing the Delivery of Pharmacy Services," *American Pharmacy* NS35, no. 1 (1995): 39–45.

5. J. McCormack et al., "Research Demonstrates Health Care and Savings Potential," *NARD Journal* March, (1996): 39–41.

6. *International Pharmaceutical Abstracts* [database online]. Bethesda, MD: American Society Health-Systems Pharmacists; 1970–present. Updated monthly. Available from University of Arkansas for Medical Sciences Medical Library; OVID Technologies, Inc., Version 3.0, release 6.2.

7. Anonymous, "Do We Have a Problem Here?" *American Druggist* November (1993): 32–33.

8. American Diabetes Association, "Standards of Medical Care for Patients with Diabetes Mellitus," *Diabetes Care* 17 (1994): 616–623.

9. M.I. Harris, C.C. Cowie, and L.J. Howie, "Self-monitoring of Blood Glucose by Adults with Diabetes in United States Population," *Diabetes Care* 16 (1993): 1,116–1,123.

10. S.L. Traub, and D. Laubenstein, 1992. Endocrine and Metabolism. In *Basic Skills in Interpreting Laboratory Data*, ed. S.L. Traub, 147–154. Bethesda, MD: American Society of Hospital Pharmacists.

11. National Diabetes Group, "Report of the Expert Committee on Glycosylated Hemoglobin," *Diabetes Care* 7 (1984): 602–606.

12. DCCT Research Group, "Diabetes Control and Complications Trial (DCCT). The Effect of Intensive Insulin Treatment of Diabetes on the Development and Progression of Long-term Complications in Insulin-dependent Diabetes Mellitus," *New England Journal of Medicine* 329 (1993): 977–986.

13. J.V. Santiago, "Lessons from the Diabetes Control and Complications Trial," *Diabetes* 42 (1993): 1,549–1,554.

14. D.E. Goldstein et al., "Is Glycohemoglobin Testing Useful in Diabetes Mellitus? Lessons from the Diabetes Control and Complications Trial," *Clinical Chemistry* 40 (1994): 1,637–1,640.

Survey used to identify diabetes cognitive services offered by pharmacies and the degree of diabetes control achieved as recorded by pharmacists

ORAL SULFONYLUREA SURVEY

Patient Information:

Demographics

patient name _____ age _____ weight _____

id# _____ sex _____ height _____

insurance plan name _____

Risk Factors (check all that apply)

❑ smoker   ❑ ethanol user   ❑ sedentary

❑ diet NOT monitored on regular basis

Concomitant Disease States (check all that apply)

❑ peptic ulcer disease   ❑ cancer   ❑ renal disease

❑ coronary artery disease   ❑ hypertension   ❑ liver disease

❑ other, please specify _____

Concomitant Medications (check all that apply)

❑ anabolic steroids   ❑ phenylbutazone

❑ b_2 adrenergic blockers   ❑ L-asparaginase

❑ phenytoin   ❑ salicylates

❑ corticosteroids   ❑ sympathomimetics

❑ ethanol containing products   ❑ sulfonamides

❑ fibric acid derivatives   ❑ thiazide diuretics

❑ pentamidine   ❑ others, please specify _____

❑ nicotinic acid   _____

❑ oral anticoagulants   _____

Diabetes Pharmacotherapy

❑ Yes   ❑ No   insulin

❑ Yes   ❑ No   dosage adjustment of insulin within past six months

❑ Yes   ❑ No   oral sulfonylurea

Outcome Indicators:

Fasting Blood Sugar Levels
date (within the last three months) _____ value (mg/dL) _____
date (3–6 months ago) _____ value (mg/dL) _____
date (6–9 months ago) _____ value (mg/dL) _____

Source for above information:
❑ patient   ❑ nurse in physician's office
❑ physician   ❑ pharmacy records
❑ other, please specify _____

Hemoglobin A_{1c}
date _____ value (%) _____
date _____ value (%) _____
date _____ value (%) _____

Source for above information:
❑ patient   ❑ nurse in physician's office
❑ physician   ❑ pharmacy records
❑ other, please specify _____

Pharmacy Information:

Demographics
pharmacist name and license number _____
pharmacy name_____
pharmacy address _____
city, state, zip _____

Cognitive Services
❑ Yes   ❑ No   Pharmacist monitors compliance of patient taking antidiabetic agents.
                        (If yes, please check all that apply)
                        ❑ patient reminded to refill prescriptions
                        ❑ dates on refills checked to verify not overdue
                        ❑ other, please specify _____
❑ Yes   ❑ No   Pharmacist counsels patients concerning use of antidiabetic agents.
                        (If yes, please check all that apply)
                        ❑ correct administration of medication
                        ❑ importance of lifestyle modifications to therapy
                        ❑ symptoms of hypoglycemia
                        ❑ symptoms of hyperglycemia
                        ❑ importance of regular monitoring of blood glucose level
                        ❑ other, please specify _____

❑ Yes   ❑ No   Pharmacist counsels patients concerning lifestyle modifications.
(If yes, please check all topics which are discussed)
    ❑ appropriate diet
    ❑ potential drug interactions between diabetic therapy and
       OTC products
    ❑ ethanol intake

❑ Yes   ❑ No   Pharmacy monitors blood levels. If yes, who monitors?
(Please check all that apply)
    ❑ pharmacist   ❑ technician
    ❑ pharmacy intern   ❑ patient
    ❑ other, please specify _____

❑ Yes   ❑ No   Pharmacy demonstrates use of blood glucose meters to patients/
caregivers
    ❑ every time a blood glucose meter is purchased
    ❑ sometimes, when patients/caregivers seem unsure
    ❑ sometimes, when patients/caregivers ask
    ❑ other, please specify _____

❑ Yes   ❑ No   Pharmacy conducts regular blood screening.
(If yes, please check all that apply)
    ❑ monthly   ❑ annually
    ❑ every three months   ❑ specific to needs of patients
    ❑ every six months   ❑ other, please specify
                           _____

❑ Yes   ❑ No   Pharmacy educates patient/caregivers on disease process of diabetes.
(If yes, please check all that apply)
    ❑ provides with written material
    ❑ pharmacist is a certified diabetes educator
    ❑ pharmacist utilizes special training skills/CE
    ❑ other, please specify _____

CHAPTER 15

Economic Evaluations and Diabetes

Dev S. Pathak, DBA and Thomas A. Burke, PharmD

Diabetes and its treatment have significant economic implications for society, as evidenced by estimated health expenditures for diabetes and its complications in the range of $85–$105 billion in the United States in 1992. With constrained resources, health care professionals need to understand the burden of any illness, benefits and costs of alternative treatments, and the process of combining benefits and costs for the purpose of comparing alternatives. The economic evaluation approach seems best suited for this task. Full and partial economic evaluation techniques will be reviewed with descriptions that have appeared in the recent diabetes literature. Key words: *cost–benefit analysis, costs and cost analysis, diabetes mellitus, economics, health expenditures, pharmaceuticals*

The current environment of health care requires demonstration of economic efficiency along with the proof of efficacy and effectiveness of alternative therapies. With constrained resources, health care professionals need to understand the burden of any illness, benefits and costs of alternative treatments, and the process of combining benefits and costs for the purpose of comparing alternatives (i.e., the process of establishing the worth of alternative treatments). Although there are many approaches for evaluating the worth of a treatment and making choices between competing treatments, the economic evaluation approach seems to be best suited for this task and is gaining in popularity in the Western hemisphere of the world. The major reason for the popularity of this approach is that economic evaluation makes decision making more explicit and decision makers more accountable to their peers, payors, and patients.[1] Hence, some of the major economic evaluation techniques will be reviewed and how they have been used in evaluating alternative treatments for diabetes will be presented.

COST OF DIABETES

A review involving some facts regarding the economic cost of diabetes to society is warranted because the following question is often asked first: what is the cost of diabetes, or any illness, to society? Unfortunately, an answer to this question varies depending on who is asking the question and what approach one uses to measure "cost." A recent study estimated the prevalence of diabetes mellitus between 31 and 45 individuals per 1,000 population, or between 3.4 percent and 4.5 percent of the U.S. population in 1992. Persons with diabetes accounted for between $85 and $105 billion in health care expenditures, which was between 11.9 percent and 14.6 percent of such expenditures in 1992. The indirect costs, such as the valuation of lost productivity to the patient, family, and friends, were not evaluated in this study.[2] However, previous research has shown that the indirect costs of diabetes are approximately equal to the direct costs, with the indirect to direct cost ratio of 1.09.[3]

The cost of diabetes can be placed in perspective when it is compared to the cost of treating persons without diabetes and the cost of other prevalent diseases. Rubin et al. reported that the ratio of total health expenditures in 1992 for persons with diabetes ($9,493 per capita) to those without diabetes ($2,604 per capita) was 3.6 to 1.0.[2] Furthermore, when the economic cost in the United States of diabetes is compared with the economic cost of cancer (total cost of $104 billion and direct cost of $35.3 billion in 1990)[4] and of depression (total cost of $43.7 billion and direct cost of $31.3 billion in 1992),[5] it seems that the direct costs of diabetes outweigh those associated with either cancer or depression. Even if differences in the cost estimates can be attributed to differences in methodologies used in calculating costs and the differences in the time periods in which these costs were calculated, it is obvious that diabetes and its treatment have significant economic implications for society.

Cost of illness and health expenditure studies, such as those discussed above, provide important information for understanding the macro implications of any therapy and are helpful in terms of overall market size estimation. However, these types of analyses are not very useful for making choices between specific competing therapies in micro settings, such as those within individual hospitals or managed care organizations. What these organizations need are incidence-based costs; information at the micro level to answer questions such as what is the relative worth of different therapies in treating and detecting the complications of diabetes? Pharmacoeconomic evaluations serve this purpose.

Pharmacoeconomic evaluation consists of comparing outcomes and costs of a pharmaceutical program or service to the next best alternative from selected perspectives. The aim of this approach is to identify, measure, value, and establish a link between both inputs (resources consumed) and outcomes so that relative worth of selected pharmaceutical programs and services can be established.

ECONOMIC EVALUATIONS

There are four Es of any economic evaluation: efficacy (can it work?), effectiveness (does it work?), equity (is it reaching those who need it?), and efficiency (is it worth doing?). Clinicians are generally familiar with terms such as efficacy, effectiveness, and equity, but not with the term efficiency as used by economists. Efficiency is the establishment of relative worth of a treatment and is a valuable tool for resource allocation decisions. It is important to remember that an analysis of efficiency cannot be superimposed on unefficacious or ineffective treatments. In other words, most efficiency studies assume that some degree of efficacy and effectiveness are already established for treatment alternatives. The second important issue is to remember that questions of equity (i.e., fairness) are usually not considered by economic evaluations. Therefore, efficiency is the focus of any economic evaluation.

Two fundamental questions are helpful in answering the question of efficiency (is it worth doing?):

1. Does the evaluation examine two or more alternatives?
2. Does the evaluation examine costs (i.e., resource expenditures), health outcomes, or both?

A full economic evaluation requires a "yes" response to both questions. By evaluating two alternatives, the relative worth of each alternative may be established. A partial economic evaluation is characterized by a "no" response to either question.[1,6] Four commonly recognized full pharmacoeconomic evaluation techniques are cost-minimization, cost-effectiveness, cost–utility analyses, and cost–benefit. This article briefly describes each full economic evaluation technique with an example of each type of analysis from the diabetes literature. Finally, the use of quality-of-life instruments in the study of diabetes is discussed before providing conclusions.

FULL ECONOMIC EVALUATIONS

Cost-Minimization Analysis

Cost-minimization analysis (CMA) is an economic evaluation technique in which the costs are measured monetarily and outcomes are proven to be identical. Costs measured in a CMA should extend beyond drug acquisition cost and should include all relevant costs, such as the cost associated with monitoring. The decision rule for this type of analysis is that the treatment with the lowest monetary cost should be selected.

Alexis et al. published a CMA, though termed a "cost impact survey," in which diabetic patients previously stabilized on glipizide (Glucotrol) were converted to glyburide (Diabeta).[7] The cost of the drug, both the acquisition cost for the Veterans Affairs (VA) Hospital and the average wholesale price, were the only costs considered. This analysis was conducted prior to generic availability of each drug, thus cost savings would differ given that both glipizide and glyburide are now available from generic drug manufacturers. The effect of each drug was assumed to be equivalent, based on comparative literature regarding the therapeutic effects of each agent. The authors assumed titration could be accomplished during routine office visits and that dosage titration would adequately reflect glycemic control of the patient. After seven months of titration, the dosage reduction from glipizide to glyburide was 47 percent, which conferred a 43 percent cost savings. The annualized cost savings for converting 211 patients from glipizide to glyburide were $15,232.02 and $17,688.81, based on average wholesale price and VA cost, respectively.

Cost-Effectiveness Analysis

Cost-effectiveness analysis (CEA) incorporates both cost and effect. Cost is measured monetarily, while effect is measured in physical units.[8] The result is a cost-effectiveness ratio, such as cost per life-year, which is calculated and used to make decisions. A strategy is more cost-effective than another strategy if it results in cost savings, with an equal or better outcome, or it has an additional benefit that is worth the additional cost. The term "cost-effective" is a relative one since a therapy cannot be considered "cost-effective" in isolation.[8,9]

Siegel et al. conducted a study on the cost-effectiveness of different screening programs for detecting diabetic nephropathy in patients with insulin-dependent diabetes mellitus (IDDM).[10] The authors used conditional probabilities to simulate the progression to renal complications in a newly diagnosed cohort of IDDM patients. Four separate strategies for detecting albuminuria were examined: a standard strategy without systematic screening, and three separate strategies with systematic screening in order of increasing aggressiveness. Program one consisted of screening the urine with Albustix®, while programs two and three used urinalysis as a screening method to detect microalbuminuria. Patients in the standard strategy group were initiated on hydrochlorothiazide upon a diagnosis of hypertension. Patients in the screening programs were started on enalapril, to delay renal function deterioration.

The standard strategy group initiated pharmacologic treatment after two of three consecutive blood pressure readings above 140/90. Patients in this group were treated with hydrochlorothiazide, eventually replaced with furosemide three years later, due to renal function deterioration. Half of the patients were diagnosed with hypertension within two years, 25 percent within three to five years, and the remaining 25 percent were never diagnosed with hypertension and never treated. The remaining three strategies instituted screening programs. Program one consisted of screening the urine with Albustix. Patients with readings (> 300 mcg/min) on two of three occasions were classified as having proteinuria and were started on enalapril. Programs two and three were more aggressive in their approach by using urinalysis as a screening method to detect microalbuminuria. Patients in program two were treated with enalapril when "significant" microalbuminuria was present (> 100 mcg albumin/mg of urine creatinine), while patients in program three were treated when microalbuminuria was present (> 20 mcg albumin/mg of urine creatinine). The ability of enalapril to impede the progression of nephropathy was estimated from reports in the literature, using a conservative estimate of a 50 percent delay and an aggressive estimate of a 75 percent delay.

In this study, cost was measured as the net health care cost of the program, while the effectiveness measure was the net improvement in life expectancy of participants. All costs were discounted at 5 percent and represent costs in the base year, 1991. The cost-effectiveness ratio was calculated discounting cost and life-years, which maintained consistency in the valuation of costs relative to the effects.

Results show that systematic screening of program one was less costly and more effective than the standard program with no screening. Thus, the standard program was eliminated as a cost-effective alternative. Programs one, two, and three were compared with incremental analysis, which is a procedure that measures the additional cost incurred to obtain each additional unit of effect from a more expensive strategy. Program three produced an additional year of life expectancy at a cost of $7,900–$16,500 when compared to program one. Program two was "dominated" by program three because it achieved fewer benefits for more cost than would be achieved if program three was applied to a fraction of the population. The authors concluded that program three resulted in the most cost-effective use of resources because the cost per year of life saved in program three compared favorably to the cost per life-year saved under other health interventions.[10] The ultimate decision as to whether the additional benefit is worth the additional cost, however, depends on the total budget available and the cut-off level of each nondominated alternative.[11]

Cost–Utility Analysis

One problem with CEA is that it does not take into account the differences in the quality of sur-vival between patients on different diabetes therapies. The most important question in diabetes therapy is, how do patients value enhanced duration vis à vis enhanced quality of life? An answer to this question is provided by calculating utility weights assigned for various health states throughout the therapy period, as in cost–utility analysis (CUA). These utility weights are then multiplied by the time spent in each health state to arrive at the amount of quality-adjusted life-years (QALY) for each patient. Then, cost per QALY ratios are calculated for each alternative measure to prioritize different treatments. Sometimes arbitrary guidelines are established for making decisions. For example, one could use a rule of thumb such as every treatment that costs $50,000 or less per quality QALY should be adopted, but a treatment that costs more than $150,000 should not be adopted.

Kiberd and Jindal compared different methods of screening for diabetic nephropathy in two groups of hypothetical IDDM patients using CUA.[12] All patients in this study were assumed to have a duration of disease of greater than five years, with relevant outcomes based on conditional probabilities incorporated into a Markov model. The study consisted of screening patients for microalbuminuria compared to screening for hypertension and macroalbuminuria. Once hypertension or albuminuria was detected, patients were placed on an angiotensin converting enzyme inhibitor to prevent progression toward end-stage renal disease.

Direct costs to the patient and insurer were the only costs included in the study. The author used the time trade-off method, described in Drummond et al.,[6] in order to obtain utility values. Utility values were calculated for present health, hypertension with medications, IDDM with blood pressure medication, functioning renal transplant, and dialysis. Incremental analysis showed that screening for microalbuminuria produced an additional undiscounted 0.1287 years compared to screening for hypertension and macroalbuminuria. When the quality of survival was taken into account using utility values, screening for microalbuminuria produced an additional 0.0097 QALYs. Based on the results, the authors concluded screening for microalbuminuria was "unproved and potentially costly."[12(p.1598)]

Cost–Benefit Analysis

Cost–benefit analysis (CBA) is an economic evaluation technique in which clinical outcomes, as well as inputs, are valued in monetary terms. The result is a cost–benefit ratio or a net monetary benefit value that is used to judge the relative value of therapies. Net benefits, with a positive dollar value indicating overall savings, are preferred as a decision rule compared to a cost–benefit ratio in CBA.[6,8] Thus, CBA captures the numerous outcomes of this study in a single measure, allowing comparisons across treatments of different diseases, something CEA is unable to accomplish. A major caveat of CBA is the requirement of the monetary valuation of human lives and quality of life. Thus, the emphasis of CBA is measuring the value of livelihood as opposed to the value of life.

A recent study by Elixhauser et al. used CBA to compare net monetary health benefits of diabetic women receiving preconception plus prenatal care compared to receiving prenatal care only.[13] The premise of the preconception care program was that achievement of optimal glycemic control prior to pregnancy would improve maternal and neonatal outcomes. A recent meta-analysis had estimated that the risk of congenital abnormalities in women receiving prenatal care only was eight-fold greater compared to those receiving preconception plus prenatal care.[14] Outcomes for both groups were estimated from a literature review and where literature review was inadequate, the incidence of outcomes was estimated by an expert panel of six physicians based on their experience. The preconception care consisted of nurses, dietitians, and social workers providing education and counseling, while physicians treated hypertension and diabetic complications of the participants.

Costs included both the direct cost of the program and the direct nonmedical cost of lost productivity by women participating in either program. The costs associated with each abnormality were evaluated with different methods. For example, costs for heart abnormalities included only the cost of the initial surgery. Other abnormalities with significant long-term costs, such as spina bifida, used lifetime direct medical costs in the cost calculation. All program and adverse outcome costs were valued at net present value. The perspective was that of the third-party payor; therefore, the indirect cost of morbidity and mortality were not included.

The net benefit of the preconception plus prenatal care compared to the prenatal care–only program was $1,720 per enrollee. When direct nonmedical costs were included in the analysis, the net benefit decreased to $1,430 per enrollee. The net benefit arose from two factors, the prevention of expensive congenital abnormalities and a decreased amount of deliveries in the preconception care group, as 12.7 percent of the women in the preconception care program decided the risks of pregnancy were too great or were advised to avoid pregnancy. The total cost calculation, therefore, was based on a differing number of deliveries per group, with 27 more deliveries in the prenatal care–only program considered. Sensitivity analysis estimated a $258–$2,504 per enrollee net benefit of the preconception care program. Finally, the managed care perspective avoided the difficulties associated with the valuation of treatment benefits, such as the avoidance of morbidity and mortality, and intangible benefits that would require valuation if the authors had chosen a societal perspective.

PARTIAL EVALUATIONS USING HEALTH-RELATED QUALITY-OF-LIFE MEASURES

Although economists prefer that full economic evaluations of treatments be used for the purposes of decision making, partial evaluations based on health-related quality-of-life (HRQOL) considerations may be extremely relevant for diabetic patients. There are many issues involved in using

HRQOL instruments in a disease state. Due to space limitations, interested readers are directed to consult a primer by MacKeigan and Pathak[15] and a book by Spilker.[16] One of the issues of interest to most clinicians is whether to use a generic or a disease-specific HRQOL instrument in measuring the impact of diabetes treatments. Generic instruments are normally designed to measure the complete spectrum of functions, disability, and disease that are relevant to HRQOL and, hence, they can be used to compare HRQOL changes across different diseases. This aspect is important when funding decisions are to be made in the public arena. Although there are many generic health status measurement instruments, three that are very popular are the Sickness Impact Profile, the Medical Outcomes Study SF-12 and SF-36, and the Nottingham Health Profile.

Several disease-specific measures have been developed for use in patients with diabetes. The rationale for developing such a measure is to focus on issues of importance to diabetics and avoid impertinent issues.[16] The diabetes quality of life (DQOL) measure was the first disease-specific diabetes measure developed. DQOL was used to assess quality-of-life outcomes for patients enrolled in the Diabetes Control and Complications Trial.[17] Although originally developed for IDDM patients, the intent of the researchers was to develop an instrument with applicability to a wide range of insulin- and non–insulin-dependent diabetics. Many other diabetes disease-specific instruments have been developed and tested. For example, Nerenz et al. published a study regarding the use of the generic SF-36 and a questionnaire on 19 diabetes-specific measures for Types I and II diabetic patients at the Henry Ford Hospital in Detroit.[18] Their experience showed that the administration of the SF-36 questionnaire was feasible in the ambulatory setting and provided useful data given the disparity of patient and physician reported scores.

•   •   •

As can be seen from this brief overview of the use of economic evaluations in diabetes and its treatments, the application of economic evaluation tools may not always result in lower cost treatments. The purpose of economic evaluation is to identify treatments that are most efficient from the resource allocation perspective. Few economic evaluations have been reported in the literature regarding pharmaceuticals or care provided by pharmacists in the treatment of diabetes and its complications. Since pharmacists have a significant role in caring for patients with diabetes, it is essential that additional research be conducted in this area. Regarding the use of HRQOL measures, the true value of the use of these evaluation tools is not in the final values obtained for making a decision, but in explicating the process used in the valuation of many subjective outcomes that cannot be adequately captured by objective outcomes.

REFERENCES

1. Z. Hakim, J.F. Pierson, and D.S. Pathak, "A Proposed Model for Conducting Institutional-Specific Cost-Effectiveness Analysis: A Case Study of Lipid-Lowering Agents." *Pharmacy Practice Management Quarterly* 16, no. 1 (1996): 78–97.

2. R.J. Rubin, W.M. Altman, and D.N. Mendelson, "Health Care Expenditures for People with Diabetes Mellitus, 1992." *Journal of Clinical Endocrinology and Metabolism* 78, no. 4 (1994): 809A–809F.

3. American Diabetes Association. *Direct and Indirect Costs of Diabetes in the United States in 1987.* Alexandria, VA: ADA, 1988.

4. M.L. Brown, "The National Economic Burden of Cancer: An Update." *Journal of the National Cancer Institute* 82, no. 23 (1990): 1,811–1,814.

5. P.E. Greenberg et al. "The Economic Burden of Depression in 1990." *Journal of Clinical Psychiatry* 54, no. 11 (1993): 405–418.

6. M.F. Drummond, G.L. Stoddart, and G.W. Torrance, *Methods for the Economic Evaluation of Health Care Programmes.* New York: Oxford University Press, 1987.

7. G. Alexis, R. Henault, and H. Sparr, "Conversion from Glipizide to Glyburide: a Prospective Cost-Impact Survey." *Clinical Therapeutics* 14, no. 3 (1992): 409–417.

8. J.M. Eisenberg, "Clinical Economics: A Guide to the Economic Analysis of Clinical Practices." *Journal of the American Medical Association* 262, no. 20 (1989): 2,879–2,886.

9. P. Doubilet, C.W. Milton, and B.J. McNeil, "Use and Misuse of the Term 'Cost-Effective' in Medicine." *New England Journal of Medicine* 314, no. 4 (1986): 253–256.

10. J.E. Siegel et al. "Cost-Effectiveness of Screening and Early Treatment of Nephropathy in Patients with Insulin-Dependent Diabetes Mellitus." *Journal of the American Society of Nephrology* 3, no. 4 (suppl.) (1992): S111–S119.

11. M.C. Weinstein, and W.B. Stason, "Foundations of Cost-Effectiveness Analysis for Health and Medical Practices." *New England Journal of Medicine* 296, no. 13 (1977): 716–721.

12. B.A. Kiberd, and K.K. Jindal, "Screening to Prevent Renal Failure in Insulin Dependent Diabetic Patients: an Economic Evaluation." *BMJ* 311, no. 7020 (1995): 1,595–1,599.

13. A. Elixhauser et al. "Cost-Benefit Analysis of Preconception Care for Women with Established Diabetes Mellitus." *Diabetes Care* 16, no. 8 (1993): 1,146–1,157.

14. C.A. Combs, and J.L. Kitzmiller, "Spontaneous Abortion and Congenital Malformations in Diabetes." *Baillere's Clinical Obstetrics and Gynaecology* 5, no. 2 (1991): 315–331.

15. L.D. MacKeigan, and D.S. Pathak, "Overview of Health-Related Quality-of-Life Measures." *American Journal of Hospital Pharmacists* 49, no. 9: 1992; 2,236–45.

16. B. Spilker, ed. *Quality of Life and Pharmacoeconomics in Clinical Trials*. Philadelphia: Lippincott-Raven Publishers, 1996.

17. The Diabetes Control and Complications Trial Research Group. "Reliability and Validity of a Diabetes Quality of Life Measure (DQOL) for the Diabetes Control and Complications Trial (DCCT)." *Diabetes Care* 11, no. 9 (1988): 725–732.

18. D.R. Nerenz et al. "Ongoing Assessment of Health Status in Patients with Diabetes Mellitus." *Medical Care* 30, no. 5 (suppl.) (1992): MS112–MS124.

Index

A

Acarbose, 53, 73–76
  anemia with, 76
  failure of, 9
  gastrointestinal adverse effects, 73–75
  hepatic transaminases, elevated, 75–76
  hypoglycemia with, 76
ACE inhibitors, 97–98
  calcium channel blockers, combination
    therapy, 30–31
  diabetic nephropathy, 28–29
Acetohexamide, 54
Alcohol, intake of, 86
Alpha-1 blockers, antihypertensive therapy, 98
Alpha-glucosidase inhibitors, 62–63
  geriatric patients, 109
Amaryl, 54
Anemia, acarbose and, 76
Angiotensin converting enzyme inhibitors. *See*
  ACE inhibitors
Antihyperglycemic agents, self-management
  education, 20–22
Antihypertensive agents, 69–78, 97–99
  acarbose, 73–76
    anemia, 76
    gastrointestinal adverse effects, 73–75
    hepatic transaminases, elevated, 75–76
    hypoglycemia, 76
  ACE inhibitors, 97–98
  adverse effects, management of, 70
  alpha-1 blockers, 98
  beta blockers, 98

  calcium channel antagonists, 98–99
  metformin, 71–73
    folate absorption, 72
    gastrointestinal adverse effects, 71
    hypoglycemia, 72–73
    lactic acidosis, 71–72
    metallic taste, 72
    vitamin B_{12} absorption, 72

B

B_{12} absorption, metformin and, 72
Beta blockers, antihypertensive therapy, 98
Biguanide, geriatric patients, 109

C

Calcium channel blockers
  ACE inhibitors, combination therapy, 30–31
  antihypertensive therapy, 98–99
  diabetic nephropathy, 29–30
Calories, intake of, 85
Carbohydrates, intake of, 85
  counting, 88
  sources of, 88–89
Case study, 111–19
Chlorpropamide, 54
Chromium, 90
Clinical practice guidelines, 124–25
Cognitive function, geriatric patients, 106
Cognitive services, diabetes, 134–36
Combination therapy, sulfonylureas,
  metaformin, failure of, 9–10

Complications
  acute, 15–17
  long-term, 17
  self-management education, 14–17
Confidant, transplant pharmacist as, 39
Control, in type II diabetes, 5–6
  study results, 6
  United Kingdom, prospective diabetes study, 5–6
Cost, of diabetes, 44, 137–43
  cost-benefit analysis, 141
  cost-effectiveness analysis, 139–40
  cost-minimization analysis, 139
  cost-utility analysis, 140–41
Counselor, transplant pharmacist as, 39

D

Delayed gastric emptying, 60–62
Designer, specialist therapy, transplant pharmacist as, 40
Diabeta, medication, 54
Diabetes mellitus, type II
  acarbose, 69–78
  antihyperglycemic agents, 69–78
  case study, 111–19
  cognitive services, 134–36
  costs of, 44
  diabetic nephropathy, 25–32
  disease state management, 123–28
  economic impact, 137–43
  geriatric patients, 103–10
  hypertension, 93–101
  metformin, 69–78
  new developments, 59–68
  nutritional guidelines, 81–91
  pharmaceutical care, impact of, 129–36
  pharmaceutical principles, 43–48
  pharmacist's role, growth of, 81–91
  self-management education, 13–24
  sulfonylureas, 51–58
  transplant patient, 33–42
Diabetic nephropathy, 25–32
  clinical course, 25–26
  combination therapy, 30–31

  management, 28–30
    ACE inhibitors, 28–29
    calcium channel blockers, 29–30
  pathogenesis, 26–27
  screening, 27–28
Diabinese, 54
Diet. *See* Nutritional therapy
Diuretics, 99
Drug interaction monitor, transplant pharmacist as, 39–40
Dual combination therapy, sulfonylureas, metaformin, failure of, 9–10
Dymelor, 54

E

Economic evaluations, 137–43
  cost-benefit analysis, 141
  cost-effectiveness analysis, 139–40
  cost-minimization analysis, 139
  cost-utility analysis, 140–41
Education
  of geriatric patients, 108
  interventions, 126
  self-management and, 13–24
    aspects of, 14–23
    complications, 14–17
      acute, 15–17
      long-term, 17
    disease state, 14–17
    foot care guidelines, 19
    goals of therapy, 17–18
    importance of, 17–18
    monitoring, pharmacologic, 20–23
    nonpharmacologic therapy, 18–20
      diet, 18
      exercise, 18–19
    patient limitations, 17
    pharmacologic therapy, 20–23
      antihyperglycemic agents, 20–22
      hypoglycemic agents, 20
      insulin administration, 21
      self-monitoring, 22
    preventive measures, 19
    risk factor reduction, 18–20
    team approach, 20

Educator, transplant pharmacist as, 39
Enzyme inhibition, 62–63
Exercise, 18–19
  in geriatric patients, 108
Extrapancreatic effects, sulfonylureas, 53–54

F

Fat, intake of, 85–86, 89–90
Fiber, intake of, 86
Folate absorption, metformin and, 72
Foot care guidelines, 19
Formulary modifications, 125–26

G

Gastrointestinal adverse effects
  acarbose, 73–75
  gastric emptying, delayed, 60–62
  metformin, 71
Geriatric patients, 103–10
  cognitive function, 106
  complications of disease, 104–5
    immunological, 105
    metabolic, 105
    neurological, 104–5
    vascular, 104
    visual, 105
  dietary changes, 106
  goals of therapy, 105–6
  insulin, 109
  lifestyle, 108
  medications, additional, 107
  monitoring, 109
  musculoskeletal abnormalities, 106
  renal function, 107
  risk factors, 103–4
  symptoms, 105
  therapy, 107–9
    nonpharmacological therapy, 107–8
      diet, 107–8
      education, 108
      exercise, 108
      lifestyle, 108
    pharmacological therapy, 108–9
      alpha-glucosidase inhibitor, 109
      biguanide, 109

  insulin, 109
  sulfonylureas, 108–9
  vision, altered, 106
Glimepiride, 54
Glipazide, 54
Glucotrol, 54
Glucotrol XL, 54
Glyburide, 54
Glynase, 54

H

Health-related quality-of-life, evaluations,
  141–42
Hepatic transaminases, elevated, with acarbose,
  75–76
Hypertension with diabetes, 93–101
  antihypertensive therapy, 97–99
    ACE inhibitors, 97–98
    alpha-1 blockers, 98
    beta blockers, 98
    calcium channel antagonists, 98–99
  diuretics, 99
  nondrug therapy, 97
Hypoglycemia
  acarbose, 76
  metformin, 72–73
  self-management education, 20

I

Immunological complications, geriatric
  patients, 105
Initial therapy
  after failure of, 7–10
  agent for, 6–7
  drug therapy, 5
Insulin administration, self-management
  education, 21
Insulin-like growth factors, 63–65

L

Lactic acidosis, with metformin, 71–72
Limitations, of patient, self-management
  education, 17

M

Management, 3–12. *See also* Pharmaceutical
  care; specific agent
  acarbose, 69–78
  antihyperglycemic agents, 69–78
  case study, 111–19
  diabetic nephropathy, 25–32
  disease state management, 123–28
  economic impact, 137–43
  geriatric patients, 103–10
  hypertension, 93–101
  metformin, 69–78
  new developments, 59–68
  nutritional guidelines, 81–91
  pharmaceutical care, impact of, 129–36
  pharmaceutical principles, 43–48
  pharmacist's role, growth of, 81–91
  self-management education, 13–24
  sulfonylureas, 51–58
  transplant patient, 33–42
Meal planning, 82–83, 87–88. *See also*
  Nutritional therapy
Metabolic complications, geriatric patients, 105
Metallic taste, with metformin, 72
Metformin, 52–53, 71–73
  failure of, 9
  gastrointestinal adverse effects, 71
  hypoglycemia, 72–73
  lactic acidosis, 71–72
  metallic taste, 72
  vitamin B$_{12}$ absorption, 72
Micronase, 54
Micronutrients, 86
Minerals, 90
Monitoring
  drug therapy, 45–47
  pharmacologic, 20–23
Musculoskeletal abnormalities, geriatric
  patients, 106

N

Nephropathy, diabetic, 25–32
  clinical course, 25–26
  combination therapy, 30–31
  management, 28–30
    ACE inhibitors, 28–29
    calcium channel blockers, 29–30

  pathogenesis, 26–27
  screening, 27–28
Neurological complications, geriatric patients,
  104–5
Nonpharmacologic therapy, 18–20
  diet, 18
  exercise, 18–19
Nutritional therapy, 18, 81–91
  alcohol, 86
  calories, 85
  carbohydrates, 85
    counting, 88
    sources of, 88–89
  chromium, 90
  fat, 85–86, 89–90
  fiber, 86
  geriatric patients, 106, 107–8
  goals of, 83–85
  meal planning, 82–83, 87–88
  micronutrients, 86
  minerals, 90
  protein, 85
    role of, 89
  sodium, 86
  sweeteners, alternative, 86
  vitamins, 90

O

Organ transplant, 33–42
  solid, success in, 34–36
  transplant pharmacist, roles of, 36–40
    confidant, 39
    counselor, 39
    drug interaction monitor, 39–40
    educator, 39
    patient care manager, 40
    patient profile manager, 40
    specialist therapy designer, 40
  for treatment of diabetes, 34
Orinase, 54

P

Pancreatic effects, sulfonylureas, 53
Pathogenesis, diabetes, 4
Patient care manager, transplant pharmacist as,
  40

Patient limitations, self-management education, 17

Pharmaceutical care, 3–12, 43–48, 59–68. *See also under* specific agent
  acarbose, 69–78
  antihyperglycemic agents, 69–78
  case study, 111–19
  costs of diabetes, 44
  current drug use process, 43
  diabetic nephropathy, 25–32
  disease state management, 123–28
  drug therapy monitoring, 45–47
  economic impact, 137–43
  geriatric patients, 103–10
  hypertension, 93–101
  impact of, 129–36
  initiation of, 5
  metformin, 69–78
  new developments, 59–68
  nutritional guidelines, 81–91
  pharmaceutical principles, 43–48
  pharmacist's role, growth of, 81–91
  relationships, 47
  resources, 47
  self-management education, 13–24
  sulfonylureas, 51–58
  transplant patient, 33–42

Pharmacist, expanding role of, 81–91

Postprandial glucose elevations, agents attenuating, 60

Pramlintide, 60–62

Preventive measures, self-management education, 19

Profile, patient, manager, transplant pharmacist as, 40

Protein
  intake of, 85
  role of, 89

Q

Quality-of-life, health-related, evaluations, 141–42

R

Relationships, in pharmaceutical care, 47

Renal function, geriatric patients, 107

Resources, pharmaceutical care, 47

Risk factor reduction, 18–20
  self-management education, 19

S

Self-management
  education, 13–24
    aspects of, 14–23
    complications, 14–17
      acute, 15–17
      long-term, 17
    disease state, 14–15, 14–17
    foot care guidelines, 19
    goals of therapy, 17–18
    monitoring, pharmacologic, 20–23
    nonpharmacologic therapy, 18–20
      diet, 18
      exercise, 18–19
    patient limitations, 17
    pharmacologic therapy, 20–23
      antihyperglycemic agents, 20–22
      hypoglycemic agents, 20
      insulin administration, 21
      self-monitoring, 22
    preventive measures, 19
    risk factor reduction, 18–20, 19
    self-management, importance of, 17–18
    team approach, 20
  importance of, 17–18

Self-monitoring, self-management education and, 22

Sensitivity, of insulin, agents increasing, 63–66

Sodium, intake of, 86

Solid organ transplantation, success in, 34–36

Specialist therapy designer, transplant pharmacist as, 40

Sulfonylureas, 51–58
  acarbose, 53
  agents, 54
    differences between, 54–56
  extrapancreatic effects, 53–54
  failure of, 7–9
  geriatric patients, 108–9
  mechanism of action, 53
  metformin, 52–53
  pancreatic effects, 53
  pathophysiology of disease, 52

Survey, diabetes cognitive services, 134–36

Sweeteners, alternative, 86

T

Taste, metallic, with metformin, 72
Team approach, self-management education
    and, 20
Thiazolidinediones, 65–66
Tolazamide, 54
Tolbutamide, 54
Tolinase, 54
Transplantation, 33–42
    solid organ, success in, 34–36
    transplant pharmacist, roles of, 36–40
        confidant, 39
        counselor, 39
        drug interaction monitor, 39–40
        educator, 39
        patient care manager, 40
        patient profile manager, 40
        specialist therapy designer, 40
Treatment, 3–12. *See also* Pharmaceutical care;
    specific agent
    acarbose, 69–78
    antihyperglycemic agents, 69–78
    case study, 111–19
    diabetic nephropathy, 25–32
    disease state management, 123–28
    economic impact, 137–43
    geriatric patients, 103–10
    hypertension, 93–101
    metformin, 69–78
    new developments, 59–68
    nutritional guidelines, 81–91
    pharmaceutical care, impact of, 129–36
    pharmaceutical principles, 43–48
    pharmacist's role, growth of, 81–91
    self-management education, 13–24

    sulfonylureas, 51–58
    transplant patient, 33–42
Type II diabetes mellitus, 3–12
    acarbose, 69–78
    antihyperglycemic agents, 69–78
    case study, 111–19
    diabetic nephropathy, 25–32
    disease state management, 123–28
    economic impact, 137–43
    geriatric patients, 103–10
    hypertension, 93–101
    metformin, 69–78
    new developments, 59–68
    nutrition therapy, 85
    nutritional guidelines, 81–91
    pharmaceutical care, impact of, 129–36
    pharmaceutical principles, 43–48
    pharmacist's role, growth of, 81–91
    self-management education, 13–24
    sulfonylureas, 51–58
    transplant patient, 33–42

U

United Kingdom, prospective diabetes study,
    5–6

V

Vascular complications, geriatric patients, 104
Vision, altered, in geriatric patients, 105, 106
Vitamins
    B$_{12}$ absorption, metformin and, 72
    intake of, 90
Voglibose, 62–63

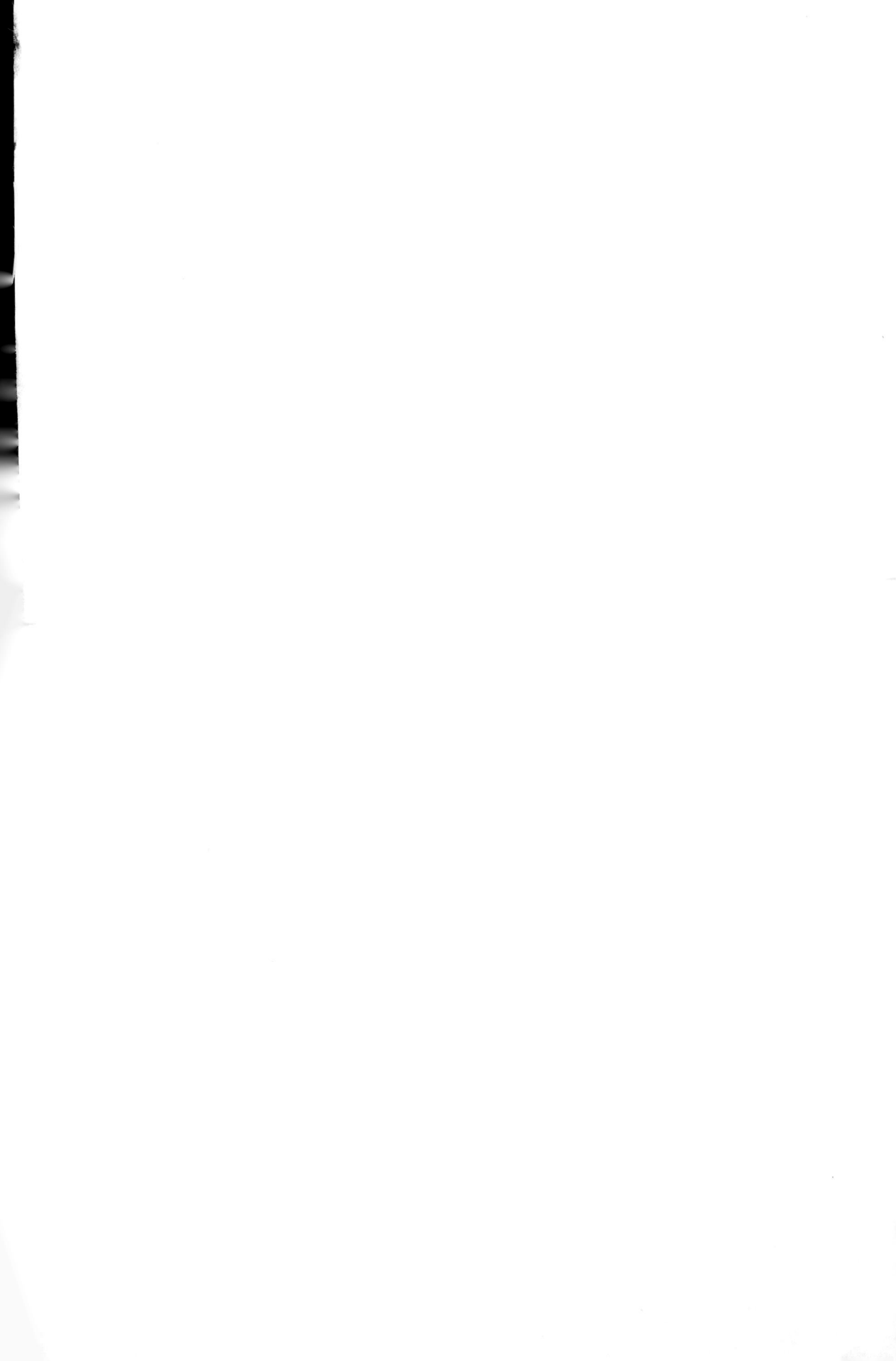

www.ingramcontent.com/pod-product-compliance
Lightning Source LLC
Chambersburg PA
CBHW081538220326
41598CB00036B/6478